# The BC Health Care Assistant Professional's Handbook

Comprehensive Practice Workbook, and BC HCA Career Roadmap



COMPLETE
TEST PREPARATION INC.
WWW.TEST-PREPARATION.CA

**We strongly recommend that students check with exam providers for up-to-date information regarding test content.**

ISBN-13: 9781772456097

Version 10 March 2026

Complete Test Preparation Inc. is an independent publisher based right here in Victoria, BC. While we've spent years in the classroom and countless hours triple-checking our questions against the provincial curriculum, we want to be clear: We are not affiliated with, endorsed by, or involved with the BC Care Aide & Community Health Worker Registry or any government health authority.

Our mission is simply to provide the best "kitchen-table" coaching and practice tools to help you succeed on your own terms. All trademarks and Registry names mentioned in this book belong to their respective owners and are used here for identification purposes only.

Published by
Complete Test Preparation Inc.
Canada
Visit us on the web at http://www.test-preparation.ca
Printed in the USA

## About Complete Test Preparation Inc.

**Why Choose Complete Test Preparation?** You want to spend your valuable study time where it counts the most. We've got you covered.

Since 2005, we have helped hundreds of thousands of students succeed with over 145 study guides and online courses. We know that tests change, which is why we keep our content current and relevant.

**Study with a Purpose** With this purchase, you are doing more than just preparing for a test. You are supporting a mission to improve education globally. We are proud to support charities that bring learning opportunities to those who need them most.

**Learn more about our mission:**
https://www.test-preparation.ca/charities-and-non-profits/

**You have definitely come to the right place.**
If you want to spend your valuable study time where it will help you the most - we've got you covered today and tomorrow.

**Thank you for studying with us!**

# Contents

# Launchpad: From Classroom to Clinic

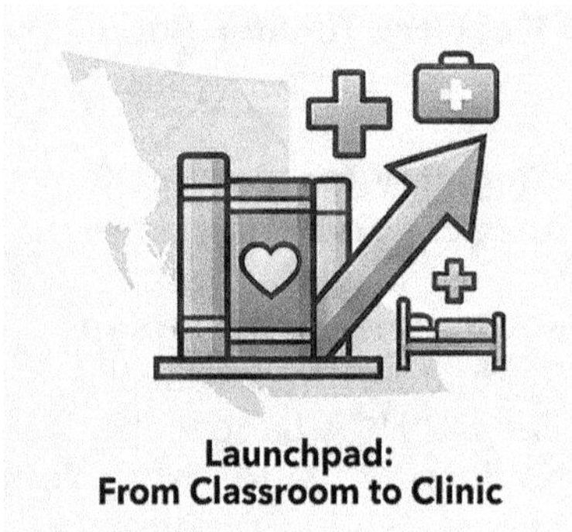


**A Note from the Team in Victoria**

You’ve got a big day coming up, and we’re glad you’re here.

Let’s be honest: nobody likes taking tests. But in British Columbia, the path to becoming a registered Health Care Assistant isn’t just about what you know—it’s about proving you’re ready to provide the high-quality care our seniors and families deserve.

Since 2005, we’ve been sitting at our desks right here in the Pacific Northwest with one goal: making sure a test doesn’t stand between you and your career. We’ve helped hundreds of thousands of students get past the “exam jitters” with guides that are hand-crafted, not mass-produced. We don’t just “utilize resources”—we roll up our sleeves and triple-check every question to make sure it matches what you’ll actually see on exam day.

Your Success Has a Reach Beyond the Classroom
When you choose a Complete Test Preparation guide, you're doing more than just hitting the books. You're helping us give back. We believe that everyone deserves a chance to learn, which is why a portion of every sale goes directly to educational charities that support "forgotten" students who need a hand up. You're getting ready for a career of helping others, and you're starting that mission right here with us.

We know how much is riding on this. Whether you're aiming for a spot in a local health authority or a community care home, we've got your back.

Thanks for trusting us with your future. Let's get to work.

Cheers,

Brian
Complete Test Preparation Inc.

## How to Tackle 200 Questions (Without Losing Your Mind)

**Let's be honest:** looking at a stack of 200 practice questions feels a lot like looking at a mountain of laundry. If you try to do it all at once, you're going to get overwhelmed, tired, and—worst of all—you'll start making "silly" mistakes that don't reflect what you actually know.

At Complete Test Preparation, we've spent years in the classroom and at the desk. Here is our "BC-grown" strategy for getting through this workbook with your sanity intact.

**1. The Power of the "15-Minute Sprint"**
Don't clear your Saturday for this. Your brain isn't built to absorb medical competencies for six hours straight. Instead, use "chunking."

**The Rule:** Set a timer for 15 minutes.

**The Goal:** Do 10 to 12 questions. That's it.

**The Reward:** When the timer dings, get up. Stretch. Grab a coffee. Fold that laundry.

**Why it works:** You'll stay sharper, and those 15-minute bursts add up fast. Four "sprints" a day means you've tackled nearly 50 questions without ever feeling burned out.

**2. The "Read It Twice" Rule**
In the heat of a test, your brain likes to play tricks. It sees a word it recognizes and jumps to a conclusion before you've even finished the sentence.

**First Read:** Read the question to understand the scenario. (e.g., "Mr. Henderson is agitated during his morning bath...")

**Second Read:** Read the question to find the specific ask. (e.g., "What is the FIRST thing the Care Aide should do?")

**The Trap:** "Big Prep" loves to include "distractor" answers that look right but don't actually answer the specific question. Reading twice is your best defense.

**3. Identify the "Who" and the "Where"**
Before you look at the multiple-choice options (A, B, C, D), identify two things:

Who is the priority? (In BC, the answer is almost always the resident's safety or dignity).

Where are you? (Are you in a long-term care facility or doing home support? The "correct" answer can change based on the setting!)

**4. Don't Fight the Questions**
Sometimes you'll hit a question that feels "unfair" or worded strangely.

Don't linger. If you don't know it in 30 seconds, circle it and move on.

**The Secret:** Often, a later question in the workbook will actually give you a hint or a "lightbulb moment" for the one you skipped.

**5. Be Kind to Yourself**

You are training for one of the most important roles in our healthcare system. You're the one who provides the hands-on care that keeps our seniors safe and happy.

If you get a question wrong, don't sweat it. That's why we provided the Rationales.

A "wrong" answer in this workbook is just a "lesson" you won't have to learn during the real exam.

# The "Core Foundation" Sets

**Mastering the Essentials of the BC Bedside**
The questions in this section cover the universal skills that every Health Care Assistant needs, regardless of where they hang their scrubs. Whether you're working the night shift in a busy Vancouver hospital or providing home support to a neighbor in Penticton, these topics are the "bread and butter" of your daily life.

**These aren't just "test topics"—they are the pillars of great care:**

**Basic Care Activities:** Understanding the "how-to" of your daily tasks.

**Person-Centred Care & Advocacy:** Keeping the resident's dignity at the heart of everything.

**Personal Care & Assistance (ADLs):** Mastering the hands-on essentials.

**Holistic Wellness:** Looking after the spirit and social life, not just the body.

**Cognitive & Mental Health Challenges:** Supporting residents with Dementia and other challenges with patience and skill.

**Interpersonal & Therapeutic Communication:** Learning how to truly hear what a resident is saying.

**Professional Practice & Ethical Boundaries:** Knowing your "Scope of Practice" and where the lines are drawn.

**Collaborative Practice:** Being the teammate every nurse wants on their ward.

The "Core Foundation" Sets

## How to Use This Section

For the best results, treat these questions with the respect they deserve. Set aside a quiet hour at the kitchen table, turn off your phone, and dive in as if this were the real deal.

**Read carefully:** "Big Prep" loves to trip people up with fast reading. Read the question twice before you pick up your pencil.

**Use the bubble sheets:** It's good practice for the mechanical side of the exam.

**The "Golden Rule" of Practice:** The goal isn't just to get a high score—it's to learn. When you're finished, don't just count your correct answers. Go to the Answer Key and read the explanations.

If you get a question wrong, don't sweat it. That's just a lesson you won't have to learn during the real exam or on your first day on the job.

**Good luck—you've got this.**

## Answer Sheet

| | A | B | C | D | E | | A | B | C | D | E |
|---|---|---|---|---|---|---|---|---|---|---|---|
| 1 | | | | | | 26 | | | | | |
| 2 | | | | | | 27 | | | | | |
| 3 | | | | | | 28 | | | | | |
| 4 | | | | | | 29 | | | | | |
| 5 | | | | | | 30 | | | | | |
| 6 | | | | | | 31 | | | | | |
| 7 | | | | | | 32 | | | | | |
| 8 | | | | | | 33 | | | | | |
| 9 | | | | | | 34 | | | | | |
| 10 | | | | | | 35 | | | | | |
| 11 | | | | | | 36 | | | | | |
| 12 | | | | | | 37 | | | | | |
| 13 | | | | | | 38 | | | | | |
| 14 | | | | | | 39 | | | | | |
| 15 | | | | | | 40 | | | | | |
| 16 | | | | | | 41 | | | | | |
| 17 | | | | | | 42 | | | | | |
| 18 | | | | | | 43 | | | | | |
| 19 | | | | | | 44 | | | | | |
| 20 | | | | | | 45 | | | | | |
| 21 | | | | | | 46 | | | | | |

**Case 1**

Your supervisor has assigned you a patient, John, a 78-year-old man with Dementia. He fell out of his bed and sprained his wrist. He is diabetic and suffers from left-sided weakness due to a stroke. He requires total care and assistance with everything he does. He has dentures. He can no longer walk alone, feed himself, bathe or dress himself, and he is incontinent of urine and stool. His vital signs are to be monitored q 4 hrs.

*1. You are preparing to shave John. You need to assemble your supplies. What is the first action that you should take?*

a. Place a warm damp towel around his face to soften his beard and relax him

b. Check the chart to see if you should shave him and if so what type of razor you can safely use.

c. Gather your towels, razor and shaving cream and proceed to John's room

d. Make certain John has the privacy required to perform ADL's

*2. You have checked the chart and it is safe to shave John using a standard razor. You should*

a. Draw the razor in the direction of hair growth

b. Draw the razor opposite the direction of hair growth

c. Pull the skin taut

d. Both a and c

**3. In performing John's daily care, you note that his toenails need to be trimmed. You should do which of the following?**

a. Gather your supplies and carefully trim his nails after cleaning his feet.

b. Ignore it

c. Note it in your documentation so that a doctor can cut his nails

d. Plan to trim his nails while you are bathing him

**4. When should you clean John's dentures?**

a. Before performing mouth care or cleaning
b. After performing mouth care or cleaning
c. Every 2 hours
d. Before and after each meal

**5. Oral care of any type should be performed**

a. At least twice per day
b. After each meal
c. Before and after each meal
d. After each meal, in the morning and each night before the patient goes to sleep

**6. To make John's bed, which of the following will you need?**

a. Gloves
b. Clean linens, gloves, and a bag for dirty linens
c. Clean linens and a bag for dirty linens
d. Clean linens

**7. When removing your contaminated gloves after making John's bed, you would**

a. Grasp the fingers of one glove using the other gloved hand and remove it

b. Grasp the cuff of one gloved had using the other gloved hand and remove it

c. Grasp the palm of one gloved hand using the other gloved hand and remove the glove leaving it in your remaining gloved hand. Then you would place your un-gloved fingers beneath the cuff of the remaining dirty glove, removing it by turning it inside out keeping the glove you have already removed inside the palm of the glove you are removing

d. Grasp the fingers of each glove and remove them by gently tugging at the ends and dispose of them in the appropriate receptacle

**8. John has gone down to radiology for a chest x-ray. You decide to take advantage of the time to make his bed. The first thing that you would do is**

a. Strip the bed of dirty linens

b. Clear the room of visitors

c. Roll the dirty linens into a ball, carry them held away from your body and deposit them in the dirty linen bag

d. Maneuver the bed into its 'flat' position

**9. The second thing that you should do in preparing to make John's bed is to**

a. Raise the bed to a comfortable working height

b. Remove the dirty linens

c. Gather your clean linens and other supplies

d. None of the above

**10. When removing the dirty linens from John's bed you would do which of the following?**

a. You should just pull them off and carry them to the dirty linen bag and place them there

b. Loosen them and roll each end toward the center and carry them to the dirty linen bag

c. Remove each item individually and inspect it for blood and then take it to the dirty laundry bag

d. It doesn't matter how you remove the linens as long as they are placed in the appropriate receptacle

**11. After removing the dirty linens, you notice that John's mattress is soiled. You should**

a. Call and have the mattress replaced

b. Document your findings

c. Wipe the mattress down

d. Make the bed and have it ready for John

**12. When preparing to make John's bed, you notice that his glasses are on the bed. You should (Choose the MOST correct answer)**

a. Remove them while making the bed and place them on the bedside table

b. Document your findings

c. Put them in your pocket so that they will not get broken

d. All of the above

**13. The following day, you are once again assigned to be John's caregiver. You are preparing to make his bed, but he cannot get up today. You must make the bed with him in it. It is best, when making an occupied bed if**

a. You can obtain assistance from a co-worker

b. You get assistance from a family member

c. Raise John's head to a 30 degree angle

d. Document that you need to make the bed while John is in it

**14. John should be bathed**

a. Daily
b. Twice daily
c. Only as needed
d. None of the above

*15. To bathe John, you will need*

a. Towels, three sheets, bath cloths, soap, warm water and a basin

b. Towels, warm water, a basin, and soap

c. Towels, wash cloths, a basin, soap and warm water

d. Towels, a warm blanket, wash cloths, a basin, soap and warm water

**16. You are going to bathe John. The MOST appropriate thing that you should do is**

a. Provide for privacy

b. Gather your supplies after making certain there is no one in the room but John

c. Gather your supplies and then provide for John's privacy

d. Bathe John as long as only family members are present

**17. Bath water should be**

a. Changed if it cools

b. Hot

c. Soapy

d. Changed between bathing of each body quadrant

**18. You have prepared to bathe John. You are now washing his arms. You should**

a. Use slow circular strokes.

b. Wash the arm proximal to distal

c. Wash the arm distal to proximal

d. Use short strokes away from the heart

**19. The taking of John's vital signs includes**

a. Temperature, blood pressure, respirations. and pulse
b. blood pressure, respirations, pulse and ROM
c. temperature, I&O, respirations, pulse and blood pressure

d. All of the above

**20. When taking John's blood pressure, you should make certain that**

a. The cuff is the correct size

b. John is lying on his left side

c. The cuff is positioned dependent to his elbow

d. The cuff is pumped to at least 20 mm above his baseline b/p

**21. You will get the most accurate temperature**

a. Under the arm

b. Rectally

c. At the groin

d. In the ear

**22. When counting the pulse rate, what points should you use?**

a. The carotid artery

b. The radial artery

c. The apical area of the heart via the chest using a stethoscope

d. All of the above

**23. While assessing John's temperature, you note that it is 101.2 degrees. What is your FIRST action?**

a. Notify your supervisor

b. Call the doctor

c. Wait the appropriate amount of time and take the temperature again

d. Have a co-worker check your work.

**24. In order that John may be placed in the sitting position in bed, you should first**

a. Check with the charge nurse to make sure the doctor allows that position

b. Ask someone to assist you in re-positioning him

c. Clear the patient's room

d. Take the patient's vital signs

**25. You have gotten a co-worker to assist you in repositioning John to a sitting position in bed. Your next action should be to**

a. Lower the bed to a comfortable working height for both you and your assistant

b. Grasp the draw sheet and count to 3, then lift/pull in the direction of the head of the bed

c. Explain to John what you are going to do

d. None of the above

**26. You have gotten a co-worker to assist you in repositioning John and you have explained to him what you are going to do. What is your next action?**

a. Lower the bed to a comfortable working height

b. Reiterate to John what you will be doing

c. Assess John's ability to assist you

d. Grasp the draw sheet, count to 3, then lift/pull toward the top of the bed

**27. John is preparing get up out of bed into a wheelchair for the first time after his admission. It is important to encourage him to sit on the side of the bed and dangle his feet for a while to ensure that**

a. Drops his blood pressure.

b. Has enough will to get up out of bed

c. Gets dizzy.

d. He can tolerate the movement.

**28. Should you decide to transport John by wheelchair, It is important to remember that you should push him from behind in all of the following scenarios except**

a. entering the elevator

b. re-entering his room

c. when you go into the cafeteria

d. when you are going down the hall

**29. When preparing to transfer John from his bed to the wheelchair you should**

a. position the chair at a 45 degree angle at his bedside

b. position the chair at a 30 degree angle at his bedside and lock the wheels

c. position the chair to a 45 degree angle at his bedside and lock the wheels

d. position the chair at a 30 degree angle at his bedside

**30. When transferring John to the wheelchair you should make certain that**

a. The wheelchair is sturdy

b. You have the chair positioned at a 43 degree angle to the bed

c. Most of the wheels are locked

d. The bed is in its lowest position

**31. When lifting, transferring or moving patients to a chair, the MOST important consideration is**

a. Comfort

b. Documentation

c. Protocol

d. Safety

**Case 2**

Paul, a 45-year-old construction worker has been admitted to the hospital for surgery. The doctor has determined that he requires an ostomy. He has been assigned to you for care.

**32. When providing ostomy care, you should**

a. Clean the area around the stoma or ostomy site thoroughly with warm soap and water

b. Avoid the ostomy area and clean all surrounding areas thoroughly

c. Obtain assistance in cleaning the ostomy area

d. Avoid the use of soap on the ostomy area

**33. An ostomy site is**

a. An opening allowing for the exit of urine from the body

b. An opening allowing for the exit of stool from the body

c. An operative site which has been closed recently requiring frequent dressing changes

d. Both a and b

**Case 3**

Joyce is a 57 year old patient who has been assigned to you. She had surgery yesterday.

**34. Joyce begins talking about the death of her sister to you. You should**

a. Listen

b. Leave the room

c. Tell her about the death of your brother

d. Advise her to talk to her doctor

**35. It is appropriate for you to share the information regarding a Joyce's status with**

a. Any one the nurse aide sees fit

b. The client's family members

c. The client's roommate

d. The staff on the next shift

**36. Joyce has developed redness and skin breakdown under her right wrist restraint. If you do not report this occurrence and report it, you are guilty of**

a. Negligence

b. Slander

c. Assault

d. Threatening a patient

**37. On entering Joyce's room, you note that a laboratory technician is attempting to perform to draw blood. He is holding Joyce's arm down forcibly while she is trying to pull away and is calling for help. The tech is guilty of**

a. Slander
b. Assault
c. Nothing
d. None of the above

**38. Joyce requires the use of the bedpan. You should**

a. Turn her on her side with knees flexed
b. Ask him to lift her hips and place the bedpan beneath his buttocks
c. Raise her head to a 30 degree angle
d. None of the above

**39. After Joyce has used the bedpan, you should**

a. Empty and rinse the bedpan and store it appropriately
b. Clean her skin with disposable wipes and dry it
c. Both a and b
d. None of the above

**40. The doctor has ordered an enema for Joyce. Which of the following do you need to assemble?**

a. Bedpan, incontinence pads, gloves, a pre-prepared enema solution or hospital approved enema equipment, and lubricating solution
b. Warm water, pads, a bedpan, gloves and an apron
c. The enema solution, lubricating jell, and incontinence pads
d. Just the enema solution

**41. You should position Joyce**

a. Supine
b. Lying on her right side
c. Lying on her left side
d. Lying on her stomach

**42. The Kubler-Ross stages of grief include**

a. Denial, anger and bargaining
b. Acceptance, bargaining and denial
c. Depression, anger, acceptance, crying and denial
d. Denial, anger, bargaining, depression and acceptance

**43. Which of the following behavior is not a sign or a symptom of anxiety?**

a. Frequent hand movement
b. Somatization
c. The client asks a question
d. The client is acting out

**44. Joyce is angry because of the addition of restraints. What skill would you use to deal with her angry outbursts?**

a. Listening
b. Advising
c. Restating
d. None of the above

**45. While dealing with Joyce's bouts of anger, she becomes belligerent and her language toward you is abusive. The proper manner in which to deal with her behavior is**

a. To remain calm
b. Walk out of the room and tell your co-worker what has occurred so that you can't be sued
c. Advise Joyce that her behavior is not acceptable
d. Both a and c

**46. A person who is _______ may indicate the desire to place an unconscious barrier between themselves and others.**

a. Avoiding eye contact

b. Yawning widely

c. Making wild gestures

d. Crossing their arms across their chest

**47. When communicating with another person, _______ is/are used to emphasize an important point, _______ can show either great interest or boredom, and _______ can express encouragement or empathy.**

a. When communicating with another person, gestures are used to emphasize an important point, posture can show either great interest or boredom, and touch can express encouragement or empathy.

b. When communicating with another person, touch is used to emphasize an important point, posture can show either great interest or boredom, and gestures can express encouragement or empathy.

c. When communicating with another person, posture is used to emphasize an important point, gestures can show either great interest or boredom, and touch can express encouragement or empathy.

d. When communicating with another person, gestures are used to emphasize an important point, touch can show either great interest or boredom, and posture can express encouragement or empathy.

**48. Which, if any, of the following statements about eye contact are false?**

a. Consistent eye contact can indicate a positive reaction to a speaker.

b. Consistent eye contact can indicate a lack of trust in the speaker.

c. The use of eye contact may be dependent on the culture of the listener.

d. None of these statements are false.

**49. _______ is a technique used to put people at ease.**

a. Speaking softly

b. Making eye contact

c. Mirroring body language

d. Leaning forward

**50. Which, if any, of these statements about body language are false?**

a. Everyone uses some form of body language to communicate.

b. Interpretations of body language are universal to all cultures.

c. The study of body language is called kinetic interpretation.

d. Indications of emotion such as smiling when happy are universal.

**51. _______ can signal a lack of interest or an unfriendly attitude and can make therapeutic communication difficult to achieve.**

a. Eye contact

b. Questioning

c. Empathy

d. Nonverbal communication

**52. If a patient asks a question that is beyond the scope of your practice, the best response would be to:**

a. Make your best guess based on what you know.

b. Tell the patient that you will find them the correct answer.

c. Change the subject.

d. Give them a book on the subject.

**53. What is the recommended method of turning off a hand faucet after washing your hands?**

a. After applying lotion
a. With a paper or cloth towel
b. After putting on surgical gloves
c. None of the Above

**54. The most important standard precaution is**

a. Treat all bodily fluids as contaminated

b. Wear gloves as much as possible

c. Only wear gloves when you think a patient is contaminated

d. Always label specimens immediately

**55. What federal agency develops and monitors standards for workplace health and safety?**

a. FDA

b. ADA

c. OSHA

d. None of the Above

**56. Influenza is caused by**

a. A fungus

b. Bacteria

c. A virus

d. Protozoa

**57. A (n) ________ ________ is a legal document filed in advance by a patient which details their wishes if they are incapacitated.**

a. Last will and testament

b. Beneficiary list

c. Advance directive

d. Funeral plan

**58. Which if any of the following statements about living wills is true?**

a. They state the type of care a patient does or does not want to receive at the end of their life.

b. They are documents in which the patient chooses a surrogate who can make healthcare decisions if they are incapacitated.

c. They demand that no extraordinary measures such as CPR, are used in an effort to revive the patient.

d. All of the above.

**59. What are the two types of advance directives?**

a. A durable power of attorney and a DNR order

b. A funeral plan and a living will

c. A life insurance policy and a durable power of attorney

d. A living will and a durable power of attorney

**60. Maintaining ____________ requires that information about a patient's current medical status, treatments and discussion of further treatment is only used for its intended purpose.**

a. Confidentiality

b. Privacy

c. Discretion

d. Autonomy

# The Bedside Mentor: Core Foundation: Answers and Analysis

The Bedside Mentor:
Core Foundation:
Explanations & Rationales

**How to Use the Bedside Mentor**
**Turning Mistakes into Mastery**

If you flip to the back of this book and only look for the letters—A, B, C, or D—you're missing out on the best part of your training. We call this section the Bedside Mentor because it's designed to do exactly what a veteran Care Aide would do on your first day of clinical: explain the why behind the action.

**Here is how to "study backward" to get the most out of every question:**

**1. Don't Just Mark it Wrong—Find the "Why"**
If you missed a question, don't just put an 'X' and move on. Read the rationale. Often, you'll find that you actually knew the material, but you missed a "BC keyword" or a specific safety priority. The rationale is there to recalibrate your "HCA Compass."

**2. The "Almost Right" Trap**
In the BC Registry exams, you'll often find two answers that look "good." The Bedside Mentor explains why one is the best. Usually, it comes down to which answer is the safest, most respectful, or most "person-centred."

**1. B**

You should always make certain a patient can be shaved and what type of razor is appropriate. If a patient is septic, it may be dangerous for the patient if you shave him at all. Shaving risks a cut that could cause issues with his already compromised immune system.

**2. D**

You should always shave in the direction of hair growth which changes depending on where you are shaving. Pulling the shin taut allows shaving with minimal risk of cutting.

**3. C**

The only person who can trim a diabetics nails is a doctor due to potential for infection.

**4. A**

The appropriate sequence when administering mouth care to a person with dentures is to clean the dentures first. Then you should perform oral care or cleaning. The dentures are then clean and ready for the patient when you have completed oral care.

**5. D**

Oral care is an essential part of appropriate nursing care. You should give oral care frequently during the day to maintain good oral health.

**6. B**

You always need gloves when removing dirty linens or performing other tasks which could bring your skin into contact with pathogens or body fluids. Clean linens and a bag for dirty laundry are essential.

**7. C**

The gloves are removed in such a manner that your skin does not come into contact with contaminated areas of the gloves and they are turned so that one is contained within the other and appropriately disposed of.

**8. D**

Unoccupied beds are always made up while in the flat

position. Doing so ensures a nice smooth bed which will not irritate the skin. Additionally, it is easier to work with a bed in the flat position than with the head or foot raised.

**9. A**
You should always observe good body mechanics when working. Raising the bed to a comfortable working height ensures less back strain.

**10. B**
Dirty linens are always rolled toward the center, keeping any contaminants contained, and placed in the dirty linen bag.

**11. C**
Part of your duties when making a bed, whether occupied or unoccupied is to make certain that everything, including the mattress, is clean.

*12. A*
The patient's belongings should always be left in the room where they can easily be located by the patient.

*13. A*
It is safer for John and will promote more efficient care if you have assistance. Shifting John for changing linens can be difficult physically for one person if the patient is unable to assist you.

**14. A**
A patient should be bathed daily and then cleaned as needed between each bath.

**15. D**
You will need clean towels, soap and water and a basin of course. You will also need a blanket to cover John for privacy and dignity and to provide warmth while you bathe him.

**16. C**
John is entitled to privacy while receiving a bath. Family members are no exception. If you wait until after you provide for privacy to gather your equipment, it may be necessary to empty the room again of visitors.

**17. A**
Water should be maintained at a comfortable temperature for bathing. It should always be changed and replaced with warm water if it cools.

**18. C**
Hands and arms are always washed distal to proximal. You should always wash from cleanest to dirtiest. The armpit is considered dirty. In addition, you should always wash the patient using strokes that lead toward the heart. This increases venous return.

**19. A**
The four components of the vital sign assessment are temperature, blood pressure, pulse, and respirations.

**20. A**
If the cuff is not the proper width for your patient, you will get a false reading on your blood pressure check.

**21. B**
The rectal temperature is taken within the body cavity and therefore yields a temperature reading closest to actual body temperature.

**22. D**
The pulse can accurately be counted using any of these areas, although for most initial assessments the radial pulse is used.

**23. C**
Always double-check your vital signs to make certain there is a valid problem.

**24. B**
When repositioning a patient, it is always in the best interest of the patient and the nurse to obtain assistance. This allows for safety for both.

**25. C**
Never attempt to perform an action for the patient without first explaining what you are going to do and how you will

be going about it.

**26. C**
The MOST appropriate answer is c. You should always allow the patient to do whatever they can to assist in their own care. Never exclude them!

**27. D**
Many things occur within the body when position is changed; blood pressure may rise or fall. The patient is most likely already weakened from having been bed bound. While the patient is sitting bedside, you can evaluate his ability to move safely.

**28. A**
A wheelchair bound patient is always turned facing outward and backed into an elevator. This prevents disorientation and dizziness on the part of the patient as well as promoting the use of good body mechanics for the nurse.

**29. C**
A 45-degree angle allows space to assist your patient in the transfer but not so much that you can't stabilize him is he slips. A 30-degree angle would be too wide to allow for control over a fall. Wheelchair wheels are ALWAYS locked.

**30. D**
The bed must be in the lowest position possible for both the safety of the patient as well as the nurse. Try to get the area we are transferring the patient from as close as possible. This will enable us to 'pivot' with John rather than manually carry him to his wheelchair.

**31. D**
The safety of both patient and nurse is foremost in the transferring of patients.

**32. A**
The skin surrounding the ostomy site must be kept clean and dry. Enzymes from exudate can erode the skin if proper care is not implemented.

**33. D**
An ostomy is used to allow for the exit of feces and urine when a patient's body can no longer perform this function normally.

**34. A**
You need to listen when your patient begins to talk about loss. It is part of your therapeutic intervention as a professional.

**35. D**
Staff members involved with your patient's care are the only ones you can share information. Giving report to the next shift is appropriate.

**36. A**
If you do not address the change in status of a patient, but rather ignore it, you are guilty of professional negligence and can be held accountable.

**37. B**
Assault is the unauthorized or forcible touching of another person.

**38. A**
When preparing to place a patient on the bedpan, you should have him/her positioned on one side with knees flexed, place the bedpan beneath the buttocks and have them roll over onto the bedpan using their flexed knees to lift their hips and position themselves comfortably on the bedpan.

**39. C**
Skin care is always provided after bedpan use to prevent tissue breakdown. You must always empty and rinse the bedpan and store it appropriately after use.

**40. A**
You would need all this equipment to perform the enema, protect yourself and the patient's linens and to lubricate the anal opening for ease of entry.

**41. C**
The patient is positioned on the left side to facilitate entry

of the enema fluid into the colon. The colon is situated within the abdomen such that the flow of the enema fluid from this position would enter the rectum flowing naturally into the descending colon and on across the transverse colon to the ascending colon.

**42. D**
The five phases of this grief model include denial, anger, bargaining, depression and acceptance.

**43. C**
If the client is asking questions, they are coping with feelings. All of the other answers are symptoms of an anxious patient.

**44. A**
To address the reason for her anger, you must listen to why she is angry.

**45. C**
It is appropriate to advise a patient that abusive behavior is unacceptable. Above all, you MUST remain calm and professional.

**46. D**
A person who is **crossing their arms across their chest** may indicate the desire to place an unconscious barrier between themselves and others.

**47. A**
When communicating with another person, gestures are used to emphasize an important point, posture can indicate either great interest or boredom, and touch can express encouragement or empathy.

**48. D**
None of these statements are false.
Consistent eye contact can indicate a positive reaction to a speaker.
Consistent eye contact can indicate a lack of trust in the speaker.

The use of eye contact may depend on the culture of the listener.

**49. C**
The idea of mirroring body language to put people at ease is commonly used in interviews. Mirroring the body language shows that they are understood.

**50. C**
The study of body language is called kinetic interpretation is false.

**51. D**
Nonverbal communication can signal a lack of interest or an unfriendly attitude, and can make therapeutic communication difficult to achieve.

**52. B**
If a patient asks a question and you do not know the answer, the best response is the response that is the most helpful. I.e. that you will help this in finding the answer. Saying that you don't know or similar responses are not helpful to the patient.

**53. B**
Turning off the tap with a paper towel prevents contamination from the tap.

**54. A**
The most important standard precaution is **to treat all bodily fluids as contaminated.**

**55. C**
The United States Occupational Safety and Health Administration (OSHA. is an agency of the United States Department of Labor. Its mission is to prevent work-related injuries, illnesses, and occupational fatality by issuing and enforcing standards for workplace safety and health.

**56. C**
Influenza, commonly referred to as the flu, is an infectious disease caused by RNA viruses of the family Orthomyxoviridae (the influenza viruses), that affects birds and mammals. The most common symptoms of the disease are chills, fever, sore throat, muscle pains, severe headache, coughing, weakness/fatigue and general discomfort.

Although it is often confused with other influenza-like illnesses, especially the common cold, influenza is a more severe disease than the common cold and is caused by a different type of virus.

**57. C**

An **advance directive** is a legal document filed in advance by a patient which details their wishes if they are incapacitated.

An advance health care directive, also known as living will, personal directive, advance directive, or advance decision, are instructions given by individuals specifying what actions should be taken for their health if they are no longer able to make decisions due to illness or incapacity, and appoints a person to make such decisions on their behalf. A living will is one form of advance directive, leaving instructions for treatment. Another form authorizes a specific type of power of attorney or health care proxy, where someone is appointed by the individual to make decisions on their behalf when they are incapacitated. People may also have a combination of both. It is often encouraged that people complete both documents to provide the most comprehensive guidance regarding their care. One example of a combination document is the Five Wishes advance directive in the United States.

**58. D**

The following are true about living wills:

They are documents in which the patient chooses a surrogate who can make healthcare decisions if they are incapacitated.
They demand that no extraordinary measures such as CPR, are used in an effort to revive the patient.

**59. D**

Two types of advance directives are **a living will and a durable power of attorney.**

An advance health care directive, also known as living will, personal directive, advance directive, or advance decision, are instructions given by individuals specifying what actions should be taken for their health if they are no longer able to make decisions due to illness or incapacity, and appoints a person to make such decisions on their behalf. A living will is one form of advance directive, leaving instructions for treatment. Another form authorizes a specific type of power of attorney or health care proxy, where the individual appoints someone to make decisions on their behalf when they are incapacitated. People may also have a combination of both. It is often encouraged that people complete both documents to provide the most comprehensive guidance regarding their care. One example of a combination document is the Five Wishes advance directive in the United States.

**60. A**

Maintaining confidentiality requires that information about a patient's current medical status, treatments and discussion of further treatment is only used for its intended purpose.

# Core Foundation Set 2

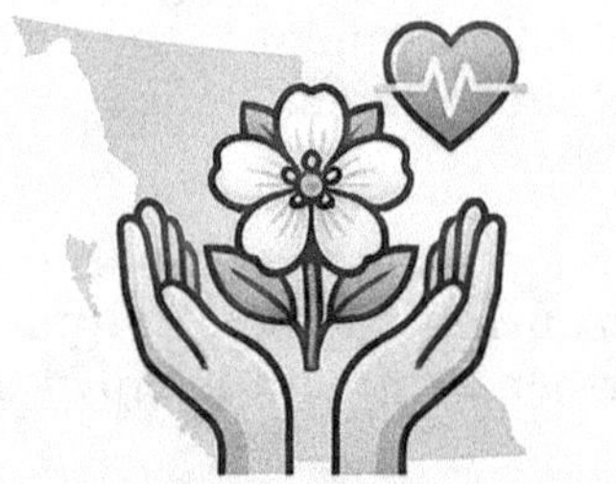

Core Foundation Set 2

**You're Building the Foundation!**
If you've just finished the first set of questions—take a breath. Whether you got them all right or found a few "stumpers," you are doing the real work. Remember, every mistake you make here in this workbook is a mistake you won't make when you're standing at the bedside or sitting in the exam room.

Many students get to this point and start to second-guess themselves. They think, "There's just so much to remember!" Here's the secret: You already have the most important tool in your kit—your common sense and your heart. When you're stuck on a question in this set, close your eyes for a second and imagine you're helping your own grandmother or a dear neighbor. Usually, the "common sense" answer is the professional one, too.

**How to approach this set:**

**Trust your gut:** Your first instinct is often the right one.

**Watch the clock:** Try to keep a steady pace, but don't rush.

**Stay curious:** If a rationale in the answer key surprises you, mark it with a star. That's your "growth zone."

You're halfway through the foundations. Keep that coffee warm, stay focused, and let's get through these next 60.

**You're doing a fine job.**

## Answer Sheet

| | A | B | C | D | E | | A | B | C | D | E |
|---|---|---|---|---|---|---|---|---|---|---|---|
| 1 | ○ | ○ | ○ | ○ | ○ | 31 | ○ | ○ | ○ | ○ | ○ |
| 2 | ○ | ○ | ○ | ○ | ○ | 32 | ○ | ○ | ○ | ○ | ○ |
| 3 | ○ | ○ | ○ | ○ | ○ | 33 | ○ | ○ | ○ | ○ | ○ |
| 4 | ○ | ○ | ○ | ○ | ○ | 34 | ○ | ○ | ○ | ○ | ○ |
| 5 | ○ | ○ | ○ | ○ | ○ | 35 | ○ | ○ | ○ | ○ | ○ |
| 6 | ○ | ○ | ○ | ○ | ○ | 36 | ○ | ○ | ○ | ○ | ○ |
| 7 | ○ | ○ | ○ | ○ | ○ | 37 | ○ | ○ | ○ | ○ | ○ |
| 8 | ○ | ○ | ○ | ○ | ○ | 38 | ○ | ○ | ○ | ○ | ○ |
| 9 | ○ | ○ | ○ | ○ | ○ | 39 | ○ | ○ | ○ | ○ | ○ |
| 10 | ○ | ○ | ○ | ○ | ○ | 40 | ○ | ○ | ○ | ○ | ○ |
| 11 | ○ | ○ | ○ | ○ | ○ | 41 | ○ | ○ | ○ | ○ | ○ |
| 12 | ○ | ○ | ○ | ○ | ○ | 42 | ○ | ○ | ○ | ○ | ○ |
| 13 | ○ | ○ | ○ | ○ | ○ | 43 | ○ | ○ | ○ | ○ | ○ |
| 14 | ○ | ○ | ○ | ○ | ○ | 44 | ○ | ○ | ○ | ○ | ○ |
| 15 | ○ | ○ | ○ | ○ | ○ | 45 | ○ | ○ | ○ | ○ | ○ |
| 16 | ○ | ○ | ○ | ○ | ○ | 46 | ○ | ○ | ○ | ○ | ○ |
| 17 | ○ | ○ | ○ | ○ | ○ | 47 | ○ | ○ | ○ | ○ | ○ |
| 18 | ○ | ○ | ○ | ○ | ○ | 48 | ○ | ○ | ○ | ○ | ○ |
| 19 | ○ | ○ | ○ | ○ | ○ | 49 | ○ | ○ | ○ | ○ | ○ |
| 20 | ○ | ○ | ○ | ○ | ○ | 50 | ○ | ○ | ○ | ○ | ○ |
| 21 | ○ | ○ | ○ | ○ | ○ | 51 | ○ | ○ | ○ | ○ | ○ |
| 22 | ○ | ○ | ○ | ○ | ○ | 52 | ○ | ○ | ○ | ○ | ○ |
| 23 | ○ | ○ | ○ | ○ | ○ | 53 | ○ | ○ | ○ | ○ | ○ |
| 24 | ○ | ○ | ○ | ○ | ○ | 54 | ○ | ○ | ○ | ○ | ○ |
| 25 | ○ | ○ | ○ | ○ | ○ | 55 | ○ | ○ | ○ | ○ | ○ |
| 26 | ○ | ○ | ○ | ○ | ○ | 56 | ○ | ○ | ○ | ○ | ○ |
| 27 | ○ | ○ | ○ | ○ | ○ | 57 | ○ | ○ | ○ | ○ | ○ |
| 28 | ○ | ○ | ○ | ○ | ○ | 58 | ○ | ○ | ○ | ○ | ○ |
| 29 | ○ | ○ | ○ | ○ | ○ | 59 | ○ | ○ | ○ | ○ | ○ |
| 30 | ○ | ○ | ○ | ○ | ○ | 60 | ○ | ○ | ○ | ○ | ○ |

**1. When performing a patient's oral care, you should first**

a. Place his head at a 45 degree angle

b. Place his head flat and have him turn his head to one side

c. Have him swish his mouth with mouthwash

d. Clean inside his mouth using gentle circular motions

**2. Patient's oral care should include**

a. Denture care

b. Gentle cleaning of the oral mucosa and lips

c. Cleaning of the tongue

d. All of the above

**3. Your co-worker tells you that the doctor has ordered cold packs for a patient's sprained wrist. You are aware that**

a. You should assess their skin before applying the pack and document your findings

b. The cold pack should be applied for no longer than twenty minutes per interval

c. You should read the order thoroughly prior to administering the cold pack.

d. All of the above

**4. After applying a cold pack, you should reassess the patient's skin**

a. Every 5 minutes

b. Every 10 minutes

c. As often as you can

d. Only after the 20 minute treatment has been completed

**5. After application of the cold pack you should**

a. Document that the order was carried out, the skin condition before and after application and the duration of the treatment

b. Document that the order was carried out and sign the chart

c. Remove the cold pack and properly dispose of it and tell your co-worker that you have completed the treatment

d. All of the above

**6. Your co-worker has rolled John onto his right side. The top sheet has been removed. To remove the bottom layers and replace them you would**

a. Roll the dirty linen from the edge of the bed inward toward John.

b. Roll the dirty linen from the top toward John's waist making certain that the dirty side is rolled toward the center then roll the remaining linen from John's feet toward the center taking the same care to keep the dirty side toward the center

c. Pull the dirty linen out from under John's body and place it in the dirty linen bag

d. Place the clean linen on top of the soiled linen and then remove the dirty linen appropriately placing in the dirty linen container

**7. Should you determine that John can help you safely, when preparing to change John's linens you would**

a. Lower the bedrail on the side opposite you leaving the other rail raised while working

b. Lower the bedrail closest to you leaving the other rail raised while working

c. Lower both bedrails while working

d. Lower the bed to its lowest position before beginning

**8. It is necessary to keep John covered while you are making his bed**

a. Only if there are others in the room
b. Always
c. If the room is cool
d. Until you get the draw sheet in place

**9. When making John's bed, you have replaced the bottom linens on your side. Your coworker is preparing to complete the change of linens. You assist John in rolling over. Your co-worker would then**

a. Grasp the roll of clean linens and unroll them from center toward the side of the bed making certain they were smooth and wrinkle free
b. Grasp the linens and pull hard so that the linens will be wrinkle free
c. Raise the bed rail
d. Place clean linens under John making certain they were wrinkle free.

**10. After you have completed making John's bed, you should wash your hands. The proper manner in which you would do this is**

a. Wash your hands using plenty of warm water and soap, thoroughly rinse and dry
b. Wash your hands, including cleaning your nails, using plenty of warm soap and water, rinse and dry
c. Wash your hands, including nails, using warm water and soap, rinse and dry
d. Wash your hands and clean your nails using warm water and soap, rinse and dry using your towel to turn off the water

**11. You should wash your hands**

a. 4 times daily
b. Before and after patient contact
c. When they become soiled
d. Both b and c

**12. You have placed a patient in a semi-sitting position. The head of his bed is at 45 degrees. This position is called**

a. Recumbent
b. Flexed
c. Sim's
d. Fowler's

**13. A patient is lying on his side with his thigh flexed. The doctor is preparing to perform a rectal examination. This position is appropriately named**

a. Fowler's
b. Freud's
c. Sim's
d. Sam's

**14. When bathing a patient, you should**

a. ALWAYS use soap, clean towels and warm water

b. Use firms strokes in the direction of the heart

c. Rub briskly with your cloth to stimulate circulation

d. Wait until later in your day because it will take a long time to bathe him

**15. When dressing a patient you should always**

a. Let him do what he can on his own and assist with what he can't do

b. Do everything for him

c. Insist that he dress himself because it is therapeutic for him to be independent

d. Get someone to assist you

**16. You have completed a patient's bath and are preparing to dress him. You have provided a clean shirt. The patient has weakness on the left side from a stoke. To put his shirt on, which arm should you put into the sleeve first?**

a. Both
b. Left
c. Right
d. Let John choose

**17. A back massage is**

a. Not a part of the bathing duties
b. The time when skin assessment can be made
c. Included in bathing
d. Both b and c

**18. Bathing is performed to**

a. Remove bacteria from the skin surface
b. Promote relaxation
c. Improve circulation
d. All of the above

**19. You are going to transfer a patient from his bed to a chair. You have placed the chair at the appropriate angle and the bed is in lowest potion. Which of the following is the BEST way to complete the transfer?**

a. Using your back and arms, pull John upright and pivot toward the chair and gently settle him into the chair
b. Wrapping your arms around John's torso and with knees slightly bent; use your legs to turn with the patient. Ask the patient, if he is capable, to grasp the arm of the chair. If now, slowly back toward the chair until you feel with your own leg that it is there. Slowly lower John into the chair.
c. Using only your arms and legs, lift the patient into your arms and settle him safely into his chair.
d. Obtain assistance from a co-worker. Each of you take one side of the patient and gently lift, using proper body mechanics, and transfer him to his chair.

**20. What is the rationale for getting a patient out of bed?**

a. To maintain muscle tone
b. To improve muscle tone
c. To allow for adequate pulmonary function
d. All of the above

**21. Which of the following is NOT a stage of assisting a patient in getting out of bed safely?**

a. Assist the patient to stand
b. Allow John to dangle his feet over the side of the bed
c. Assist John in moving to the chair
d. Asking a family member to explain to John what you are about to do

**22. Which would you do first when assisting a patient out of bed?**

a. Assist him to a standing position

b. Allow him to dangle his feet over the edge of the bed

c. Move the chair out of his way

d. Obtain the chair from across the room

**23. A patient is being transferred to a chair. You and a co-worker are helping him. Which part of your anatomy should be MOST involved in the transfer?**

a. Legs
b. Back
c. Arms and shoulders
d. Both b and c

**24. If the patient begins to become off balance or unstable during the transfer, you should**

a. Attempt to stabilize the patient by bracing him against you and guide the patient to the bedside or chair, if possible.
b. If a fall begins to occur, guide him slowly toward the floor.
c. Move back and allow the patient to slide to the floor and call for assistance
d. Both a and b

**25. If a fall occurs, as you gently glide your patient to the floor you should**

a. Protect his head
b. Protect his IV
c. Protect his drains
d. Protect his extremities

**26. After a patient's fall, the first thing that you**

**should do is**

a. Call for assistance in getting John off the floor and into bed or his chair
b. Just pick him up and complete the move
c. Assess for injuries and call for assistance
d. Talk to your assistant about what went wrong

**27. After a patient's fall, what document must you fill out?**

a. And incident report
b. The I & O sheet
c. Charting of the people who witnessed the fall
d. The vital sign flow sheet

**28. While walking by a co-worker, you overhear her telling another worker that you have not addressed a patient's restraint care in your documentation. You are aware that this is untrue and that you have done all that you should do for your patient. Your co-worker's behavior is an example of**

a. Slander
b. Assault
c. Defamation
d. Both a and d

**29. After coming on duty later in the course of a patient's care, you note that her restraints have been tied to the bed frame. You are aware that this can cause injury to the patient and is inappropriate use of her restraints. This is an example of**

a. Assault
b. Negligence
c. Appropriate action
d. Slander

**30. You have just walked into a patient's room and you overhear a lab technician telling her to allow him to draw her blood or he will tighten her restraints. The lab tech is guilty of**

a. Slander
b. Threatening a patient
c. Acting in the patient's best interest
d. Violation of Joyce's privacy

**31. Restraints may be used**

a. To force her to obey doctor's orders no matter what
b. Only at night
c. In accordance with doctor's orders only
d. None of the above

**32. All of the following are inappropriate within the scope of the hospital setting EXCEPT**

a. Documentation
b. Providing for patient privacy
c. Talking about a co-worker
d. Using gloves

**33. A patient has become confused and her doctor has ordered wrist restraints. All the following are true of restraints except**

a. They should allow as much freedom of movement as possible
b. They should be removed periodically
c. Their application should be documented
d. They should be tied to the bed frame

**34. The patient has attempted to get out of bed and has managed to slip despite her wrist restraints. The doctor orders the addition of ankle restraints. You know that**

a. The use of restraints on all four extremities is also termed 'four point restraints'
b. Range of motion exercises should be performed regularly
c. You should observe for skin breakdown
d. All of the above

**35. Prior to application of the patient's ankle restraints, she kicked the side rail bruising her knee and causing minor swelling. The doctor has ordered that a cold pack be applied to the area. You would know that**

a. The cold pack will help with swelling and pain as well as bruising
b. You should leave the cold pack in place no longer than 20 minutes
c. You should assess the skin prior to applying the cold pack
d. All of the above

**36. Before you apply the patient's cold pack, you assess her skin integrity, temperature and color. You note that the skin is extremely cold, blue-black in color in an area extending beyond the damaged originally damaged area, the tissue is extremely swollen and Joyce is complaining of intense pain. You should**

a. Not apply the cold pack until you have reported your findings to the charge nurse or doctor
b. Go ahead and apply the cold pack
c. Initiate a CODE BLUE
d. Gently massage the area before applying the cold pack

**37. While assessing John's temperature, you note that it is 101.2 degrees. What is your FIRST action?**

a. Notify your supervisor
b. Call the doctor
c. Wait the appropriate amount of time and take the temperature again
d. Have a co-worker check your work.

**38. You can count respirations while**

a. Taking John's b/p
b. Counting John's pulse
c. Taking his temperature
d. None of the above

**39. When assessing a patient's respirations you should**

a. Count the number of times his chest rises and falls in one minute
b. Auscultate his chest
c. Observe whether John is breathing easily or seems to be having difficulty
d. All of the above

**40. If a patient's 3 year old granddaughter was visiting and was watching you take her grandfather's vital signs and became curious about how you would take hers, you might explain to her that**

a. You would do it on the arm but with a smaller cuff
b. You would do it on her thigh but with a smaller cuff
c. You would do it on her ankle using a smaller cuff
d. All of the above.

**41. You came on duty at 7 A.M. It is now 1 P.M. Assuming everything is normal, how many times should you have assessed John's vital sign status?**

a. Twice
b. Once
c. PRN

d. Not at all

**42. After assessing a patient's vitals, the MOST proper way to document them would be**

a. Bp140/72, Pulse regular and bounding, Respirations 16 and shallow, temp. 99.0
b. Temp 99.0 orally, BP 140/72, Pulse regular, Respirations 16
c. Pulse regular and bounding, Temp. 99.0 orally, B/P140/72, Respirations 16 and shallow
d. None of the above

**43. When taking a rectal temperature you will need**

a. Gloves and lubricant
b. An oral thermometer
c. A rectal thermometer
d. Both a and c

**Case 3**

Joyce is a 57 year old patient who has been assigned to you. She had surgery yesterday. She has mentioned the loss of a family member to you several times.

**44. In reviewing the care that you have administered to Joyce today, you are aware that her anger may have been**

a. A stage of grief
b. Caused by her dislike of you
c. Caused by a hereditary disease
d. Temporary insanity

**45. To assist Joyce in accepting the loss of her family member you must**

a. Read everything on death and dying before approaching her
b. Be willing to talk with her about death

c. Not bring up her loss, no matter what
d. Distract her with conversation about other things

**46. James, a 19-year-old college student has been admitted to the hospital for sports injuries sustained during a hockey game. He has been assigned to you. When you enter his room to take him his breakfast tray, he comments on your appearance and tries to touch you. You should**

a. Tell him that his actions are inappropriate
b. Ignore him
c. Slap his hand
d. Call for help

**47. After telling James that his actions are inappropriate, he apologizes and you leave the room. You should**

a. Document the occurrence and your response
b. Call the police
c. Talk to your co-workers to obtain support
d. Ignore the incident

**48. Joyce's family has been in to visit her. They have told her that her sister was killed in an automobile accident. While performing her care, you note that she is silent and withdrawn. You would know that this she is experiencing which of the Kubler-Ross stages of grief?**

a. Acceptance
b. Denial
c. Bargaining
d. Depression

**49. _______ is restating something that a patient has said, usually in fewer words and with emphasis on the main points of their statement.**

a. Attending
b. Paraphrasing
c. Clarifying

d. Perception checking

**50. Facial expression, posture and tone of voice are elements of _______.**

a. Open-ended questions
b. Nonverbal communication
c. Orientation process
d. Good manners

**51. Which, if any, of the following statements about nonverbal communication are true?**

a. Nonverbal communications are less reliable that verbal communication

b. Nonverbal communications remain the same, regardless of ethnicity or culture.

c. Nonverbal communications always send a clear message.

d. Nonverbal communications can emphasize or contradict verbal messages.

**52. _______ provides encourages the patient to continue talking without showing agreement or disagreement.**

a. Smiling
b. Leaning forward
c. Nodding
d. Paraphrasing

**53. Using phrases that address a person's feelings, such as "You must be worried about your headaches," demonstrates _______.**

a. Empathy
b. Interest
c. Acceptance
d. Recognition

**54. When dealing with elderly patients, always _______.**

a. Use their first names to establish intimacy.

b. Direct your questions to their caregivers.

c. Speak loudly and distinctly.

d. Address them as Miss, Mrs., or Mr., followed by their last name.

**55. When interviewing a patient with a hearing loss, remember to _______.**

a. Speak slowly and look directly at the patient.

b. Ensure that the room is brightly lit.

c. Write down your questions and have them write their answers.

d. Both a. and b).

**56. A/an _____________ is a form that is filled out as soon as possible following an event such as an injury to a patient.**

a. Tort

b. Occurrence statement

c. Testimonial

d. Incident report

**57. Using neutral remarks such as, "I see" and "I hear what you're saying" show _______ to the patient.**

a. Empathy

b. Recognition

c. Understanding

d. Avoidance

**58. If a patient refuses to make eye contact, you may find that they are _______.**

a. From a culture that considers direct eye contact rude.

b. Very tired.

c. Lying about their symptoms.

d. Disinterested in the conversation.

**59. When communicating with non-English speaking patients, professionals should:**

a. Repeat sentences word-for-word if the patient does not understand.

b. Use their children as interpreters.

c. Raise the volume of their voices.

d. Immediately employ the services of an interpreter.

**60. Which, if any, of the following statements about geriatrics are false?**

a. Geriatrics is a branch of medicine in which the focus is health care for the aging population.

b. Geriatrics differs from gerontology, which is the study of the aging process itself.

c. A geriatrician's practice is limited to persons over the age of 65.

d. None of the above.

# The Bedside Mentor: Core Foundation (Set 2)

The Bedside Mentor:
Core Foundation (Set 2)

**Reflecting on the "Heart of Care"**
You've made it through the second 60 questions! This set probably felt a little different—maybe a bit more about "judgment calls" and "communication" than just simple tasks. That's because as a BC Care Aide, your most important tool isn't your blood pressure cuff; it's your ability to read a room and a resident.

**How to Use These Explanations:**
Don't just look for the green checkmark. If you missed a question in this set, it's likely because of a "distractor"—an answer that looks mostly right but isn't the best choice for the resident's dignity or safety.

**1. The "Why" is the Win**
In this section, the rationales focus on the Holistic Wellness model. If you got a question wrong about a resident's mood or social life, read the explanation to see how we balance physical safety with emotional health.

**2. Look for the "BC Keyword"**
In our province, we use specific language like Responsive Behaviours or Informed Consent. If you see these terms in the rationales, circle them! These are the words the Registry examiners are looking for.

**1. A**
Always place the head at this angle to prevent choking.

**2. D**
Mouth care includes all areas of the mouth both inside and out.

**3. D**
You never take an order from another person. Always check the chart yourself and read the order. You should assess skin integrity at every opportunity, especially with diabetics. Cold packs are NEVER left in place longer than 20 minutes.

**4. B**
You should always reassess skin 10 minutes after the application of a cold pack.

**5. A**
You should always document after a procedure is carried out. Note everything that you can about the area of treatment both before treatment is performed and afterward.

**6. A**
Always roll dirty linen toward the center to contain contaminates.

**7. B**
Lowering the rail nearest you allows you to work and leaving the opposite rail raised provide for John's safety by preventing a fall from the bed.

**8. B**
You should always keep a clean sheet, blanket or bath blanket over the patient even when replacing top linens. This is done to provide for warmth and privacy.

**9. A**
The linens are already under John, the bedrail should already be down, and you do not pull hard on linens that a patient is lying on as this could injure the patient.

**10. D**

You would use the paper towel utilized to dry your hands to turn off the water avoiding contamination of your clean hands.

**11. D**

Hand washing is a critical part of patient care and personal safety.

**12. D**

Fowler's positioning is considered to be an upright position of varying degrees.

**13. C**

Sim's position is a side lying position with the patient's thigh flexed. This position facilitates access to the rectum and vagina for examination.

**14. B**

You can't always use soap, especially with geriatric patients. You should ALWAYS use strokes that travel in the direction heading toward the heart as this increases venous return.

**15. A**

Allowing John to do what he can promotes independence and dignity in a difficult situation. Offer assistance when needed.

**16. B**

When a patient has weakness in an extremity, that extremity is always dressed first.

**17. D**

A gentle back massage is part of the bathing process and allows inspection of the skin on the back and buttocks as well as documentation and reporting of any adverse findings.

**18. D**

The removal of bacteria, relaxation and improved circulation are all benefits of bathing.

**19. B**

None of the other answers take into account the proper use of body mechanics except for answer d. Answer d is incorrect because this exercise involves a one on one move....not an assisted move.

**20. D**

It is critical, if proper functioning of body systems is to be secured, that movement be encouraged when feasible. Extended time as a bed-bound patient impairs normal system functioning.

**21. D**

You should be the one explaining what is happening to John.

**22. B**

You must allow John to dangle his feet over the edge of the bed for a short time. This allows for settling of equilibrium, blood pressure changes to settle, and blood flow to extremities time to alter.

**23. A**

Carry the majority of the force of the move on your legs. This prevents damage to the nurses back, arms and shoulders. All play a role in the transfer, but carry the bulk of the weight on your legs.

**24. A**

Should a fall begin to occur, your first priority is to protect the patient. Stabilize him with your body by bracing him against you and if it is impossible to avoid a fall then your only alternative is to guide him, gently to the floor.

**25. A**

The correct answer is to protect John's head. IV's, drains and extremities are all important, but a head blow could be very serious, even lethal.

**26. C**

Of course, you will need assistance in getting him off the floor, but your first priority is in ascertaining whether John has sustained injuries due to the fall. You should

NOT move him further without both assistance and assessment.

**27. A**
Whenever an unexpected occurrence happens which involves a patient, or even a worker, you MUST fill out an incident report.

**28. D**
Your co-worker has spoken about you to others and the things said were untrue and could damage your reputation and endanger your license.

**29. B**
Properly trained medical personnel know that a hospital bed is created to move. Tying restraints to the bed will injure a patient at some point when the position of the bed is changed and must be avoided.

**30. B**
The tech has threatened Joyce with action he is not authorized to perform and which may cause her fear and anxiety to elicit her cooperation. This is inappropriate behavior.

**31. C**
Forcing a patient to do anything using restraints constitutes abuse and negligence. You must only use restraints in accordance with her doctor's orders.

**32. C**
Talking about a co-worker can constitute slander and defamation of character. At the least, it is unprofessional conduct and you should avoid.

**33. D**
A, b, and c are all true of the appropriate use of restraints. Tying the restraint off to the bed frame places the patient in jeopardy if the position of the bed is changed.

**34. D**
You always perform ROM exercises on restrained limbs regularly and the potential for skin breakdown is in-

creased with the addition of restraints. The term ‘four point restraints’ is indicative that four extremities have been restrained.

**35. D**

Cold packs are extremely therapeutic in the treatment of bruising, swelling and pain, however you should continually assess the patient’s skin during their use and they should be limited to an application time not to exceed 20 minutes per treatment. The skin should then be reassessed and proper documentation performed.

**36. A**

For a minor injury, you should not see these symptoms. Blue-black tissue, intense pain and extremely cool skin could indicate a blood clot or more serious tissue damage than was originally thought. You should report your findings to the proper authority.

**37. C**

Always double-check your vital signs to make certain there is a valid problem.

**38. C**

While the thermometer is registering John’s temperature, it is a good time to count his respirations. This is an example of good time management.

**39. D**

The respiratory assessment should ALWAYS include the number of respirations, the quality of them and accompanying breath sounds.

**40. D**

A child of this age could have her b/p assessed on any of the above-mentioned areas using a child’s cuff.

**41. A**

Within the 6 hours you have been on duty, given that you are to assess his vital signs every 4 hours, you should have documented them twice.

**42. B**

When noting vital signs you must give as much information as you have been able to obtain. This should include the count, quality, and anything abnormal.

**43. D**

An oral thermometer is never used to take a rectal temperature. Gloves, lubricant and a rectal thermometer are the appropriate implements utilized during this phase of vital signs.

**44. A**

Anger is one of the stages of grief and Joyce has just experienced the loss of a loved one.

**45. B**

You must be willing to talk to her about death. At some point, this is something that any patient who experiences a loss will do.

**46. A**

Setting boundaries for sexual conduct in the workplace is important.

**47. A**

You should always document harassment of any kind as well as your response. It is your protection. Remember, if you don't document, it NEVER happened.

**48. D**

Joyce is exhibiting symptoms of withdrawal and silence. She is not talking, actively grieving, or crying.

**49. B**

Paraphrasing is restating something that a patient has said, usually in fewer words and with emphasis on the main points of their statement.

**50. B**

Facial expression, posture and tone of voice are elements of nonverbal communication.

**51. D**
Nonverbal communications can emphasize or contradict verbal messages is the only statement that is true.

**52. C**
Nodding provides encourages the patient to continue talking without indicating agreement or disagreement.

**53. A**
Using phrases that address a person's feelings, such as "You must be worried about your headaches," demonstrates empathy.

**54. D**
Always address older patients Miss, Mrs., or Mr., followed by their last name. Addressing older patients by their first name may offend.

**55. A**
When interviewing a patient with a hearing loss, remember to speak slowly and look directly at the patient.

**56. D**
In a health care facility, such as a hospital, nursing home, or assisted living, an incident report or accident report is a form that is filled out to record details of an unusual event that occurs at the facility, such as an injury to a patient. The purpose of the incident report is to document the exact details of the occurrence while they are fresh in the minds of those who witnessed the event. This information may be useful in the future when dealing with liability issues stemming from the incident.

Generally, according to health care guidelines, the report must be filled out when possible following the incident (but after the situation has been stabilized). This way, the details written in the report are as accurate as possible.

Most incident reports that are written involve accidents with patients, such as patient falls. However, most facilities will also document an incident in which a staff member or visitor is injured.

If an incident involves a patient, the patient will often be monitored for a period of time following the incident (for it may happen again), which may include taking vital signs regularly. 3

**57. C**

Using neutral remarks such as, “I see” and “I hear what you’re saying” indicates understanding to the patient.

**58. A**

If a patient refuses to make eye contact, you may find that they are from a culture that considers direct eye contact rude.

**59. D**

If the patient has ‘no’ English at all, which is a little rare but does happen, then using an interpreter is the best choice. If the patient has ‘a little’ English, then speak slowly and carefully. Raising your voice will not help.

**60. C**

A geriatrician’s practice is limited to persons over the age of 65 is false. Geriatrics is a sub-specialty of internal medicine and family medicine that focuses on health care of elderly people. It aims to promote health by preventing and treating diseases and disabilities in older adults. There is no set age at which patients may be under the care of a geriatrician, or physician who specializes in the care of elderly people. Rather, this decision is determined by the individual patient’s needs, and the availability of a specialist.

# The BC Registry Insider

## Provincial Standards & Regulation Set 1

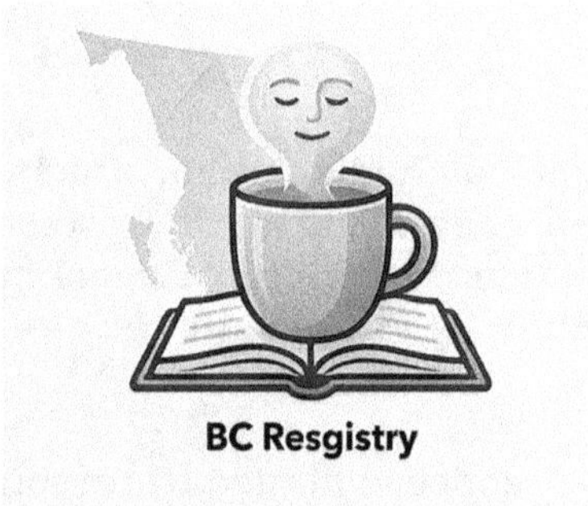


**Part 2: The BC Registry Insider**
**From "Care Aide" to "BC Registered Professional"**
You've built a rock-solid foundation in the first half of this book. Now, it's time to put on your "BC Lens."

In British Columbia, we do things a little differently than the rest of the country. We have our own Ministry of Health mandates, our own Registry requirements, and a very specific way of handling everything from "delegated tasks" to "workplace safety." This section is designed to make sure you aren't just "good at the job," but that you are Registry-Ready.

**In this first set of 45 BC-specific questions, we are going to focus on the "Rules of the Province," including:**

**The BC Care Activities Chart:** Knowing exactly what you can (and cannot) do without a Nurse's supervision.

**WorkSafeBC Standards:** Mastering the specific "Point of Care" risk assessments that keep you and your residents safe.

**The BC Care Aide Registry:** Understanding your legal obligations as a registered health professional in this province.

**Provincial Ethics & Legislation:** Navigating the Adult Guardianship Act and the Freedom of Information and Protection of Privacy Act (FOIPPA).

**A Note from the Kitchen Table**
I've seen students who are brilliant at the bedside struggle with these questions because they "overthink" the bureaucracy. Don't let the big words like "Legislation" or "Mandate" scare you off.

At the end of the day, these BC rules are just a formal way of making sure we all provide the same high level of care from Victoria to Fort St. John. When you're answering these, ask yourself: "Does this follow the BC Ministry's goal of safe, respectful, person-centred care?" If the answer is yes, you're likely on the right track.

**How to Tackle This Set:**

**Spot the "BC Keywords":** Look for terms like Informed Consent, Least Restrictive, and Collaborative Care.

**Scope is Everything:** Pay close attention to questions about what an HCA is allowed to do. In BC, we are very clear about where the HCA role ends and the Nurse's role begins.

**The Registry Mindset:** Answer these as if you are already a Registered HCA. You aren't a student anymore; you're a professional colleague.

**Take a deep breath. You've done the work—now let's get you registered.**

## Answer Sheet

| | A | B | C | D | E | | A | B | C | D | E |
|---|---|---|---|---|---|---|---|---|---|---|---|
| 1 | ○ | ○ | ○ | ○ | ○ | 26 | ○ | ○ | ○ | ○ | ○ |
| 2 | ○ | ○ | ○ | ○ | ○ | 27 | ○ | ○ | ○ | ○ | ○ |
| 3 | ○ | ○ | ○ | ○ | ○ | 28 | ○ | ○ | ○ | ○ | ○ |
| 4 | ○ | ○ | ○ | ○ | ○ | 29 | ○ | ○ | ○ | ○ | ○ |
| 5 | ○ | ○ | ○ | ○ | ○ | 30 | ○ | ○ | ○ | ○ | ○ |
| 6 | ○ | ○ | ○ | ○ | ○ | 31 | ○ | ○ | ○ | ○ | ○ |
| 7 | ○ | ○ | ○ | ○ | ○ | 32 | ○ | ○ | ○ | ○ | ○ |
| 8 | ○ | ○ | ○ | ○ | ○ | 33 | ○ | ○ | ○ | ○ | ○ |
| 9 | ○ | ○ | ○ | ○ | ○ | 34 | ○ | ○ | ○ | ○ | ○ |
| 10 | ○ | ○ | ○ | ○ | ○ | 35 | ○ | ○ | ○ | ○ | ○ |
| 11 | ○ | ○ | ○ | ○ | ○ | 36 | ○ | ○ | ○ | ○ | ○ |
| 12 | ○ | ○ | ○ | ○ | ○ | 37 | ○ | ○ | ○ | ○ | ○ |
| 13 | ○ | ○ | ○ | ○ | ○ | 38 | ○ | ○ | ○ | ○ | ○ |
| 14 | ○ | ○ | ○ | ○ | ○ | 39 | ○ | ○ | ○ | ○ | ○ |
| 15 | ○ | ○ | ○ | ○ | ○ | 40 | ○ | ○ | ○ | ○ | ○ |
| 16 | ○ | ○ | ○ | ○ | ○ | 41 | ○ | ○ | ○ | ○ | ○ |
| 17 | ○ | ○ | ○ | ○ | ○ | 42 | ○ | ○ | ○ | ○ | ○ |
| 18 | ○ | ○ | ○ | ○ | ○ | 43 | ○ | ○ | ○ | ○ | ○ |
| 19 | ○ | ○ | ○ | ○ | ○ | 44 | ○ | ○ | ○ | ○ | ○ |
| 20 | ○ | ○ | ○ | ○ | ○ | 45 | ○ | ○ | ○ | ○ | ○ |
| 21 | ○ | ○ | ○ | ○ | ○ | 46 | ○ | ○ | ○ | ○ | ○ |
| 22 | ○ | ○ | ○ | ○ | ○ | 47 | ○ | ○ | ○ | ○ | ○ |
| 23 | ○ | ○ | ○ | ○ | ○ | 48 | ○ | ○ | ○ | ○ | ○ |
| 24 | ○ | ○ | ○ | ○ | ○ | 49 | ○ | ○ | ○ | ○ | ○ |
| 25 | ○ | ○ | ○ | ○ | ○ | 50 | ○ | ○ | ○ | ○ | ○ |

## WHMIS 2015 & Infection Control

**1. Under WHMIS 2015, which of the following is a primary requirement for a workplace label on a decanted cleaning solution?**

a. The name of the manufacturer and their head office address
b. A reference to the Safety Data Sheet (SDS) for further information
c. The expiry date of the original chemical concentrate
d. The specific chemical formula and molecular weight

**2. A Care Aide is about to clean a spill and sees a symbol consisting of a flame inside a red diamond. What does this indicate about the product?**

a. It is a biohazardous infectious material
b. It is an oxidizing gas that feeds existing fires
c. It is a flammable material that can ignite easily
d. It is corrosive to metals and human skin

**3. While assisting a resident with a morning wash, you notice the basin is cracked and leaking. You find a replacement basin, but it is covered in a fine layer of dust in the supply closet. According to BC infection control "Routine Practices," what is the correct action?**

a. Wipe the basin with a dry paper towel since it hasn't been used
b. Rinse the basin with hot tap water for 30 seconds
c. Clean and disinfect the basin according to facility protocol before use
d. Use the basin as is, provided it is used for the same resident

**4. You are assigned to help a resident who has been**

**placed on "Droplet Precautions" due to a suspected respiratory infection. Which of the following sets of Personal Protective Equipment (PPE) is required before entering the room?**

a. Gloves and a gown only
b. Surgical mask and eye protection (googles or face shield)
c. N95 respirator and double gloves
d. No PPE is required as long as you stay two metres away from the bed

**5. You accidentally splash a concentrated floor disinfectant on your forearm while refilling a bucket. After immediately rinsing the area with cool water, what is your next priority according to WHMIS 2015 protocols?**

a. Finish the cleaning task so the floor isn't a slip hazard
b. Call the manufacturer listed on the bottle for medical advice
c. Check the Safety Data Sheet (SDS) for specific first aid measures
d. Apply a thick layer of antibiotic ointment and cover with a bandage

## The "No-Lift" Policy

**6. What is the primary goal of the "No-Lift" policy implemented in BC healthcare facilities?**

a. To reduce the time it takes to transfer residents between units
b. To eliminate the need for manual lifting to prevent musculoskeletal injuries (MSIs)
c. To ensure that all residents are ambulatory and can walk on their own
d. To decrease the number of staff required to work on a night shift

**7. According to WorkSafeBC, which device is considered a "mechanical lift" under the No-Lift policy?**

a. A standard manual wheelchair
b. A fixed overhead ceiling lift
c. A wooden transfer board
d. A pair of non-slip socks

**8. You are about to transfer a resident from their bed to a chair. The care plan states they are a "Mechanical Lift" transfer, but the resident insists they feel strong enough to stand with your help today. What is the correct action?**

a. Support the resident under their armpits and perform a manual stand-pivot transfer
b. Follow the care plan and use the mechanical lift as specified
c. Ask a second HCA to help you manually lift the resident to respect their wishes
d. Allow the resident to stand on their own while you wait by the chair

**9. While preparing to use a floor lift (Sling Lift), you notice a small 2 cm fray on one of the leg straps of the sling. What should you do?**

a. Use it for this one transfer and report it at the end of your shift
b. Use it only if the resident weighs less than 150 lbs
c. Remove the sling from service immediately and report the damage
d. Double-knot the frayed area to reinforce the strap before use

**10. A "Point-of-Care Risk Assessment" (PCRA. must be performed by the HCA at what frequency?**

a. Once every month during the supervisor's check-in
b. Only when a new resident is admitted to the facility
c. Before every single transfer or handling task performed
d. Only if the resident has a history of aggressive behaviour

## Cultural Safety & Humility

**11. A coworker says, "I don't see race; I treat all my residents the same." Why is this approach considered a barrier to Cultural Safety in BC?**

a. It is a helpful way to ensure everyone receives equal care
b. It ignores the unique historical and systemic barriers that Indigenous people face in healthcare
c. It is the fastest way to complete daily tasks and morning care
d. It is actually the core requirement of the BC Care Aide Registry

**12. You notice an Indigenous resident becomes quiet and avoids eye contact when you ask questions about their pain level. Based on cultural safety training, you should:**

a. Assume they are not in pain and move on to the next resident
b. Repeat the question louder and more slowly to ensure they understand
c. Allow for silence, use a gentle tone, and recognize that eye contact may be a sign of respect rather than a lack of engagement
d. Document that the resident is "uncooperative" or "non-communicative"

**13. When an HCA practices "Self-Reflection" as part of Cultural Humility, they are primarily:**

a. Looking in a mirror to ensure their uniform is clean and tidy
b. Examining their own biases and how their position of power might affect the client
c. Reciting the facility's mission statement before their shift
d. Memorizing the names of all the First Nations in British Columbia

**14. A resident's family asks if a traditional "Smudging" ceremony can be performed for their loved one who is nearing the end of life. You know the facility has a strict "No Smoking/No Burning" policy. What is the most culturally safe action?**

a. Tell the family it is illegal in BC to burn anything inside a healthcare building
b. Suggest they go outside to the parking lot to perform the ceremony
c. Advocate for the family by asking the nurse or administrator about the facility's specific "Smudging Protocol" or designated sacred space
d. Inform the family that spiritual needs are only handled by the facility's priest or chaplain

**15. You are assisting an Indigenous resident who attended a Residential School. They become visibly distressed and fearful when they see your white uniform and hear a firm, authoritative tone of voice. This is likely an example of:**

a. A personal dislike of the HCA's personality
b. Age-related dementia that makes them confused about their surroundings
c. Intergenerational trauma and a response to a healthcare system that has historically caused harm
d. A "Common Trap" where the resident is just trying to avoid having a bath

**16. Which term best describes the HCA's ability to recognize that their own cultural background may influence how they provide care to a resident?**

a. Cultural Blindness
b. Cultural Humility
c. Cultural Imposition
d. Cultural Assimilation

**17. A resident follows a Halal diet. Which of the following food items must be strictly avoided when serving their meals?**

a. Shellfish and bottom-feeding fish
b. Beef that has been prepared by a licensed butcher
c. Pork and any products containing lard or gelatin from swine
d. Caffeinated beverages and carbonated sodas

**18. You are helping a Sikh resident with their morning care. You notice they wear a small wooden comb (Kangha. in their hair and a metal bracelet (Kara). They ask you not to remove these items. What is the correct action?**

a. Explain that all jewellery must be removed for safety and hygiene reasons
b. Respect the resident's request and ensure the items remain with them as part of their faith
c. Wait until the resident is asleep to remove the items and place them in the bedside drawer
d. Inform the resident that the facility policy only allows wedding bands

**19. A Hindu resident has a dietary restriction of "No Beef." During lunch, the main course is beef stew. The resident is hungry and asks for a bowl. What should the HCA do?**

a. Serve the stew but tell the resident to leave the meat chunks in the bowl
b. Remind the resident of their religious restriction and refuse to serve them any lunch
c. Check the care plan for an alternative protein and consult with the kitchen to provide a vegetarian or chicken-based meal
d. Give the resident the stew since they asked for it, as resident choice always comes first

**20. You are caring for a Muslim resident during the month of Ramadan. The resident expresses a wish to fast from sunrise to sunset. What is the HCA's first responsibility?**

a. Force the resident to eat breakfast to ensure they can take their morning medications
b. Tell the resident that fasting is not permitted in a long-term care setting
c. Report the request to the nurse (LPN/RN) so the care team and dietitian can adjust meal and medication timings
d. Ignore the request and place the standard meal tray in front of them at the usual time

**21. Which of the following is an example of an "objective" observation that an HCA must report?**

a. The resident seems to be in a grumpy mood today
b. The resident has a raised, red rash on their left upper arm
c. The resident says they feel like they are getting a cold
d. The resident appears to be lonely because no one visited

**22. When an HCA observes a "Change of Status" in a resident, what is the most appropriate first step in the reporting process?**

a. Wait until the end of the shift to write it in the communication book
b. Call the resident's family to update them on the change
c. Verbally report the observation to the regulated nurse (LPN or RN) immediately
d. Ask another HCA if they think the change is important enough to mention

**23. While performing morning care, you notice a new 2 cm purple bruise on a resident's hip that was not there yesterday. The resident is on blood thinners. What is your priority action?**

a. Apply a warm compress to the area to help the bruise fade
b. Document the bruise in the daily flow sheet and check it again tomorrow
c. Report the new bruise to the LPN immediately, as it may indicate internal issues
d. Ask the resident if they remember falling out of bed during the night

**24. A resident who is normally alert and oriented suddenly becomes confused and is unable to remember which room is theirs. Their skin feels hot to the touch. What should you do?**

a. Lead them back to their room and suggest they take a nap
b. Give them a glass of water and wait one hour to see if the confusion clears
c. Report these symptoms to the nurse immediately as they may indicate a UTI or infection
d. Document "resident was confused today" in the chart and continue with your rounds

**25. You are assisting a resident with a meal when they suddenly begin to cough persistently and their voice becomes "wet" or gurgly. What is the most likely cause and the required action?**

a. They are bored with the food; offer a different dessert
b. They are experiencing aspiration; stop the meal and notify the nurse immediately
c. They have a dry throat; encourage them to take a large gulp of water
d. They are talking too much; tell them to sit quietly until they finish eating

**26. Which of the following is a "Do" of professional documentation in a BC care home?**

a. Use a pencil so you can erase mistakes and keep the chart tidy
b. Document care immediately after it is completed, never before
c. Use plenty of white-out to correct errors in the permanent record
d. Include your personal opinion on why a resident is acting out

**27. Which of the following is considered an "objective" (fact-based. statement for a progress note?**

a. The resident was very happy during the music therapy session
b. The resident ate 50% of their beef stew and drank 200 mL of water
c. I think the resident's daughter is upset because she didn't say hi
d. The resident was being difficult and refused to wear their blue shirt

**28. Review this "sloppy" note: "Resident was grumpy this morning and didn't want to get up. I think he is getting a cold because he looked tired." Which part of this note is objective?**

a. Resident was grumpy
b. didn't want to get up
c. I think he is getting a cold
d. he looked tired

**29. You are documenting a resident's fall. Which entry is the most professional and follows "best practices"?**

a. Resident fell because the floor was slippery; my supervisor was mad
b. Found resident sitting on the floor beside the bed at 0200. No visible injuries. LPN notified
c. The resident fell again; they really need to be more careful
d. Resident had a clumsy moment and ended up on the floor. I put them back in bed

**30. Review this note: "Mrs. Smith was very rude to me during her bath. She yelled for no reason. She is clearly depressed." What is the main "Don't" illustrated in this documentation?**

a. It uses too many medical terms
b. it is too short and lacks detail
c. It uses subjective, judgmental language and makes a diagnosis (depressed)
d. It doesn't mention the temperature of the bathwater

## Palliative & End-of-Life Care

**31. What is the primary role of a Health Care Assistant (HCA. when a resident is exploring or undergoing Medical Assistance in Dying (MAiD)?**

a. Explaining the legal criteria for eligibility to the family
b. Providing high-quality comfort care and emotional support
c. Administering the medication prescribed by the physician
d. Witnessing the formal written request for the service

**32. In British Columbia, which professional is legally permitted to perform the assessment and administration for MAiD?**

a. A Registered Care Aid with advanced palliative certification
b. Only a Registered Nurse or Licensed Practical Nurse
c. A Medical Practitioner (Doctor) or Nurse Practitioner
d. The Director of Care at the residential facility

**33. A resident you have cared for consistently tells you, "I'm tired of the pain; I want to ask about that doctor-assisted dying." What is your best response?**

a. Tell the resident you will bring them the necessary forms to sign immediately
b. Share your personal or religious views on the topic to help them decide
c. Inform your supervisor or the nurse that the resident has expressed interest in MAiD
d. Explain that as an HCA, you are not allowed to discuss the topic at all

**34. While providing morning care, a family member asks you if the MAiD procedure is "painful for the loved one." How should you handle this inquiry?**

a. Provide a detailed medical explanation of the drugs used in the process
b. Comfort the family member and refer their clinical questions to the nurse or doctor
c. Tell them not to worry because the government regulates the process strictly
d. Share a story about another resident's experience with the procedure

**35. A resident who has been approved for MAiD asks you to stay in the room and hold their hand during the final process. According to BC standards, what should you do?**

a. Politely decline, as HCAs are legally barred from being in the room
b. Stay and provide supportive presence if you are comfortable and it is permitted by your facility
c. Leave the room immediately, as your job ends once the "medical" part begins
d. Tell the resident that only family members are allowed to be present

**36. What is the primary reason for performing frequent mouth care for a resident in the final stages of life?**

a. To ensure the resident can still enjoy solid foods
b. To prevent the mouth and lips from becoming dry and painful
c. To reduce the risk of the resident developing a secondary infection like pneumonia
d. To follow standard facility protocols for morning and evening hygiene

**37. Which of the following is a common physical sign that a resident has entered the "final hours" of the dying process?**

a. An increase in appetite and sudden alertness
b. Rapid, deep breathing with a consistent rhythm
c. Skin that feels warm and appears flushed or red
d. Changes in breathing patterns, such as long pauses between breaths

**38. You are providing care for Mrs. Chen, who is actively dying. Her breathing has become noisy and moist, often called the "death rattle." Her daughter is at the bedside and is visibly distressed by the sound. What is your best response?**

a. Tell the daughter that her mother is choking and you need to call for a suction machine immediately
b. Explain to the daughter that this is a normal part of the body slowing down and usually doesn't cause the resident distress
c. Advise the daughter to leave the room for a few minutes until the sound stops
d. Suction the back of Mrs. Chen's throat vigorously to clear the sound for the family

**39. A resident in the palliative stage is experiencing significant "mottling" on their feet and lower legs. What is the most appropriate comfort measure for the HCA to take?**

a. Rub the legs vigorously with scented lotion to improve circulation
b. Apply a heating pad directly to the mottled areas to warm the skin
c. Ensure the resident is kept warm with a light blanket and avoid unnecessary friction to the skin
d. Elevate the legs above the level of the heart to reduce the discolouration

**40. While performing mouth care for a resident who is no longer conscious, you notice their mouth is clamped shut. How should you proceed?**

a. Use a tongue depressor to force the mouth open to complete the cleaning
b. Skip the mouth care entirely to avoid agitating the resident
c. Use a moistened swab to gently clean the lips and the outer gums without forcing the mouth open
d. Wait until the nurse can administer a sedative before attempting mouth care again

## Mental Health & Cognitive Impairment

**41. What is the primary goal of the "Gentle Persuasive Approach" (GPA. when working with residents who have dementia?**

a. to eliminate all forms of responsive behaviours through medication
b. to use physical force only when a resident is attempting to leave the building
c. to understand that a person's response is a result of a disease and to respond with respect and safety
d. to ensure the resident follows the facility schedule strictly to reduce confusion

**42. The term "sundowning" refers to which common occurrence in residents with dementia?**

a. a significant improvement in memory during the evening hours
b. an increase in confusion, restlessness, and agitation as the daylight fades
c. a medical requirement for residents to be asleep by sunset
d. the tendency for residents to want to go outside only during the day

**43. Mr. Henderson is standing at the secured unit door, pulling the handle and stating, "I need to get to the bus stop or I'll be late for work." What is the best initial response using a gentle persuasive approach?**

a. Tell him he is retired and doesn't have a job anymore
b. Remind him that the door is locked for his own safety and he cannot leave
c. Acknowledge his need to go to work and ask him to tell you about his job while walking with him
d. Block the door with your body and call for security to escort him to his room

**44. It is 4:00 PM, and Mrs. Grewal is becoming increasingly agitated, pacing the hallways and crying. She says she needs to go home to cook dinner for her children, who are now actually adults. How should the HCA respond?**

a. Show her a calendar and her ID to prove she lives at the care facility
b. Offer her a simple, familiar task like folding napkins or towels to help "prepare" for a meal
c. Tell her that her children already ate and don't need her help
d. Place her in a wheelchair with a lap belt so she doesn't tire herself out from pacing

**45. While you are trying to help a resident with a "sundowning" episode, they become physically aggressive and try to grab your arm. What is the safest body positioning according to Gentle Persuasive principles?**

a. Stand directly in front of the resident to show you are in charge
b. Stand at a 45-degree angle (the supportive stance) at a respectful distance
c. Move in close and hug the resident to calm them down with touch
d. Turn your back to the resident to show you are not a threat

# The BC Registry Insider: Answers and Analysis

## Thinking Like a BC Professional

The BC Registry Insider: Explanations & Standards

Welcome to the "Expert" level of your study. If you've just finished the first set of BC-specific questions, you might have noticed that the language changed a little. We've moved away from general "good ideas" and into the specific Mandates and Competencies that the BC Ministry of Health and the Care Aide Registry expect from you every single day.

In this section of the Bedside Mentor, we aren't just looking at the "right" answer—we're looking at the "Provincially Approved" answer.

**How to Use the BC Insider Key:**

**1. The "Scope of Practice" Filter**

In British Columbia, the line between an HCA and an LPN is very clear. If you got a question wrong about a task (like wound care or medication), read the rationale carefully. It will explain exactly where your "Independent" role ends and where "Supervision" begins according to BC standards.

**2. Identifying "Reportable Incidents"**

A big part of being a BC Registered HCA is knowing when to speak up. The explanations in this key highlight the BC Patient Safety & Quality Council standards. Use these to learn exactly what constitutes a "reportable event" in a BC Health Authority.

**3. Indigenous Cultural Safety & Humility**

You likely saw questions regarding cultural safety. In BC, this is a core competency. Our rationales explain why certain approaches are required to provide respectful care to Indigenous residents and their families. This isn't just "politics"—it's the law of the land in BC healthcare.

**4. The WorkSafeBC Lens**

Many of the "Correct" answers in this set are dictated by WorkSafeBC. If a rationale mentions a "Point of Care Risk Assessment" (PCRA), pay attention! That is a term you will use every single shift once you're on the ward.

**A Note from the Kitchen Table:** Some of these regulations can feel a bit like "alphabet soup"—VCH, VCHA, FOIPPA, HCAP. Don't let the acronyms get to you. These rules exist to protect you just as much as they protect the resident. When you follow the BC Standards, you're covered, you're professional, and you're providing the best care in the country.

## WHMIS 2015 & Infection Control

**1. B**
A workplace label requires the product name, safe handling instructions, and a statement that an SDS is available.

Option A is for supplier labels. Option C is rarely required on decanted labels. Option D is too technical for a standard workplace label.

💡 **Test Tip:** Remember that workplace labels are about safety and resources, not the manufacturing history of the chemical.

**2. C**
The flame pictogram identifies products that are fire hazards (flammable).

Option A uses the "trefoil" symbol. Option B (Oxidizer) is a flame over a circle. Option D (Corrosive) shows liquid pouring onto a hand and metal.

**3. C**
In a healthcare setting, any equipment that has been sitting in storage must be cleaned and disinfected to prevent the spread of environmental contaminants.

Options A and B do not meet the standard of "disinfection" required for patient care equipment. Option D is incorrect because "same resident" use still requires clean equipment.

**4. B**
Droplet precautions (used for flu or pertussis) require a mask and eye protection because droplets travel through the air but fall quickly.

Option A is for Contact precautions. Option C is for Airborne precautions (like TB). Option D is a safety risk; PPE is required upon entry.

**5. C**

The SDS is the legal document that contains specific first aid, fire-fighting, and accidental release measures for that specific chemical.

Option A ignores personal injury. Option B is too slow. Option D may cause a reaction with the chemical still on the skin.

## The "No-Lift" Policy

**6. B**

The policy is designed to eliminate manual lifting of the weight of a person to prevent back and shoulder injuries (MSIs) which are the #1 cause of lost time for HCAs in BC.

Options A and D are administrative/efficiency goals, not safety goals. Option C is a medical outcome, not a policy goal.

**7. B**

Mechanical lifts include ceiling lifts, floor/sling lifts, and sit-stand lifts.

Wheelchairs (A and transfer boards (C are assistive devices but not "mechanical lifts" that bear the full weight. Non-slip socks (D. are personal protective items.

**8. B**

The care plan is a legal document based on a professional assessment. Deviating from it, even at the resident's request, risks injury to both of you.

Options A and C involve prohibited manual lifting. Option D is unsafe if the resident is assessed as requiring a lift.

**Test Tip:** "The care plan is the boss." Unless you perform a PCRA and find the resident is worse than the care plan says, you stick to the plan or call a supervisor.

**9. C**

Slings are overhead lifting equipment. Any sign of wear or damage (fraying, tearing) makes them unsafe and they must be tagged and removed immediately.

Options A and B take a "risk it" approach which is never allowed. Option D is an unauthorized and dangerous modification.

**10. C**

A resident's status can change in an hour (fatigue, medication, confusion). You must assess the situation every time you touch the resident.

Options A, B and D are too infrequent and ignore the "in-the-moment" nature of safety.

## Cultural Safety & Humility

**11. B**

This is the "Common Trap." "Treating everyone the same" ignores the fact that people start from different places. True safety requires acknowledging identity and history.

**Test Tip:** In BC exams, "equality" (treating everyone the same) is usually wrong; "equity" (giving people what they specifically need. is usually right.

**12. C**

In many Indigenous cultures, avoiding eye contact is a sign of respect for an authority figure or Elder. Silence is often used to process thoughts.

Option B is condescending. Option D is a harmful label that misinterprets a cultural norm.

**13. B**

Cultural Humility is about looking inward to see how our own background and the "power" of our healthcare uniform might intimidate a client.

It is not about physical appearance (a. or rote memorization (c/d).

**14. B**
Most BC health authorities now have specific policies to allow smudging (which uses a very small amount of smoke) because it is a human right.

Option A is a "Common Trap"—people often cite "fire codes" to block Indigenous practices, but the HPOA and human rights laws generally provide exceptions for ceremonies.

**15. C**
Residential School survivors often have deep-seated trauma related to uniforms, bells, and strict authority. This is a "trauma-informed" care realization.

Option D is a dismissive stereotype that prevents the HCA from providing compassionate, safe care.

**16. B**
Cultural Humility involves self-reflection and the recognition of power imbalances, acknowledging that the HCA's own culture is not the "default."

Option A is ignoring culture. Option C is forcing one's own culture on others. Option D is the expectation that a resident should give up their culture to fit in.

**17. C**
Halal dietary laws prohibit the consumption of pork and any derivatives (like gelatin or lard. from swine.

Option A (Shellfish) is a Kosher restriction, not Halal. Beef (Option b. is allowed if it is slaughtered according to Halal standards.

**18. B**
The "5 Ks" of the Sikh faith (including the Kangha and Kara. are deeply sacred. Unless they pose an immediate, documented life-safety risk that cannot be mitigated, they stay with the resident.

Options A and D use "Big Prep" corporate-style rigid rules that violate human rights and person-centred care. Option C is a violation of trust and resident rights.

**19. C**

In BC, we balance "Resident Choice" with "Safety and Care Planning." If a resident asks for something against their known religious practice, we provide a safe alternative and consult the team.

Option A still involves cross-contamination of the broth. Option B is punitive. Option D is a "Common Trap"—while choice is important, impulsive requests that violate long-standing religious identity should be handled with a care-team consultation to ensure the resident isn't confused.

**20. C**

Fasting during Ramadan is a core religious duty for many Muslims. The care team must work together to ensure the resident's health (hydration, meds) is maintained during non-fasting hours.

Options A and B are culturally unsafe and ignore the resident's spiritual rights. Option D is a failure in the duty to report.

## Observation & Reporting

**21. B**

Objective observations are facts that can be seen, heard, felt, or smelled (signs). A rash is a visible, measurable sign.

Options A and D are interpretations/opinions (subjective). Option C is a "symptom" (what the resident says), not an observation made by the HCA.

**22. C**

HCAs are the "eyes and ears." Any change in status must be verbally communicated to the regulated supervisor immediately to ensure timely intervention.

Waiting until the end of shift (Choice A. is dangerous. HCAs generally do not update families on clinical changes (Choice B). Coworkers (Choice D. cannot provide clinical direction.

**23. C**
For residents on anticoagulants (blood thinners), a new bruise can signal a serious internal bleeding issue. It is a priority report.

Applying heat (Choice A. can worsen bleeding. Waiting (Choice b. is unsafe. Questioning the resident (Choice D. is helpful but does not replace the need to notify the nurse.

**24. C**
Sudden confusion (delirium) and fever in the elderly are classic signs of a Urinary Tract Infection (UTI) or other acute illness.

Napping (Choice A. or waiting (Choice b. allows the infection to worsen. Simple documentation (Choice D. without verbal reporting is a failure of duty.

**25. B**
A "wet" voice and persistent coughing during or after swallowing are "red flags" for aspiration (food/liquid entering the lungs).

Forcing more water (Choice C. or ignoring it (Choices A and D. can lead to aspiration pneumonia or choking.

## Documentation "Do's and Don't's

**26. B**
Documentation must be a chronological record of what happened. Documenting before care (pre-charting) is illegal and unsafe.

Erasable pens (Choice A. and white-out (Choice C. are strictly forbidden in medical records. Opinions (Choice D. have no place in a professional chart.

**27. B**

Facts are measurable and observable. 50% and 200 mL are specific, objective data points.

Happiness (Choice A), being upset (Choice C), and being difficult (Choice D. are all subjective interpretations of behavior.

**28. B**

"Didn't want to get up" is an observable action (the resident stayed in bed).

"Grumpy," "tired," and "I think he is getting a cold" are all subjective opinions or guesses.

**29. B**

This note is objective (sitting on the floor), provides a time, notes an observation (no visible injuries), and identifies the action taken (LPN notified).

Options A and D are judgmental or "blaming." Option d uses unprofessional language like "clumsy moment."

**30. C**

Terms like "rude" and "for no reason" are judgmental. An HCA cannot diagnose a resident with "depression."

The issue isn't the length or medical terms; it's the lack of objectivity.

## Palliative & End-of-Life Care

**31. B**

The HCA's role is always centered on the "person," not the "procedure." Providing comfort and emotional support is the core of HCA work.

Choice A is incorrect because HCAs do not provide legal or clinical eligibility advice.

Choice C is incorrect because HCAs never administer MAiD medications.

**32. C**
Under BC law and federal Bill C-7, only a physician or nurse practitioner can assess and provide the service.

Choice B is incorrect; while RNs/LPNs can assist, they cannot be the primary "provider."

Common Trap: Option B is the trap. Many students assume all nurses can "perform" it, but the law specifically identifies the "provider" as a doctor or NP.

**33. C**
Communication is key. You must ensure the resident's request is heard by the clinical team.

Choice A is incorrect because HCAs do not handle the formal documentation.

Choice D is incorrect; you can discuss it by listening and referring, you just can't act on it.

**34. B**
This respects the HCA's role as a communicator while staying within the scope of practice regarding medical information.

Choice A is incorrect; this is a "medical" explanation outside the HCA's scope.

Choice D is incorrect; this violates resident confidentiality.

**35. B**
There is no law in BC that forbids an HCA from being present for emotional support if the resident wishes it and the staff member is comfortable.

Choice A is incorrect; there is no such legal "bar" for presence, only for "participation" in the medical act.

**36. B**
Mouth care is strictly for comfort. Residents at this stage often breathe through their mouths, leading to extreme dryness.

Choice A is incorrect because most residents in the final stages are no longer eating solids.

Choice C is incorrect; while true in general care, the priority in palliative care is comfort over long-term infection prevention.

**37. D**
Irregular breathing (Cheyne-Stokes) or long pauses (apnea. are classic signs of the final hours.

Choice A is incorrect; while a "rally" can happen, a decrease in appetite is the norm.

Choice C is incorrect; skin usually feels cool and looks mottled (purple/blue) as circulation fails.

**38. B**
The "death rattle" is caused by secretions the resident can no longer swallow. It sounds worse to the family than it feels to the resident.

Choice A is a Common Trap. Suctioning is rarely used in the final hours because it is invasive and often causes more distress/secretion production.

Choice D is incorrect for the same reason—it's too aggressive for comfort care.

**39. C**
Mottling is a sign of failing circulation. The skin is fragile.

Choice A is incorrect; vigorous rubbing can tear the skin.

Choice B is incorrect; decreased circulation makes the resident highly susceptible to burns from heating pads.

**40. C**
You never force anything in palliative care. You do what is possible for comfort without causing trauma.

Choice A is incorrect and can cause injury.

Choice B is incorrect; you should still try to provide some moisture to the lips/outer mouth.

**41. C**

The GPA is built on the philosophy that a person with dementia is a person first, and their behaviours are often a response to environmental or internal triggers they can't express.

Choice A is incorrect; the goal is not "elimination" through drugs.

Choice D is incorrect; strict schedules often increase agitation in dementia.

**42. B**

This is the textbook definition of sundowning.

Common Trap: Option D. It sounds plausible because it involves time of day, but it doesn't address the psychological "confusion" element.

**43. C**

Validation and redirection are the gold standards. You meet them in their reality (work) and move them away from the door naturally.

Choices A and B are incorrect; "Reality Orientation" often causes more distress and "catastrophic reactions" in dementia.

**44. B**

Giving a resident a meaningful, familiar task ("procedural memory") can satisfy the urge to be productive and redirects the agitation.

Choice D is incorrect; a lap belt is a physical restraint and is highly regulated/restricted in BC.

**45. B**

The 45-degree angle (supportive stance) is less threatening to the resident and protects the HCA's vital organs and balance.

Choice A is incorrect; this is a "confrontational" stance.

Choices C is incorrect; touch can be misinterpreted as an attack when a resident is agitated.

# British Columbia Provincial Standards & Regulation Set 2

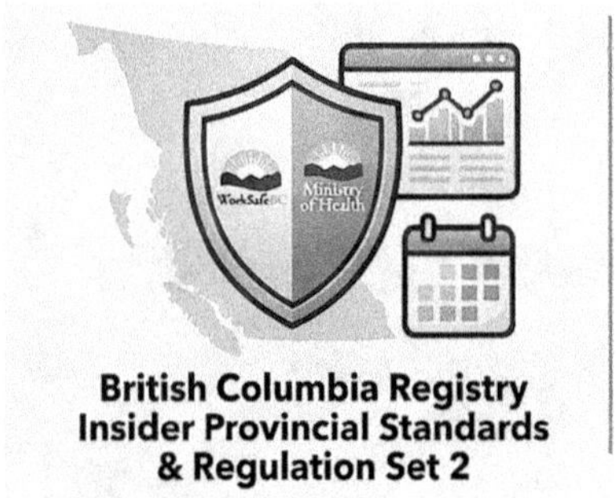

## Answer Sheet

| | A | B | C | D | E | | A | B | C | D | E |
|---|---|---|---|---|---|---|---|---|---|---|---|
| 1 | ○ | ○ | ○ | ○ | ○ | 21 | ○ | ○ | ○ | ○ | ○ |
| 2 | ○ | ○ | ○ | ○ | ○ | 22 | ○ | ○ | ○ | ○ | ○ |
| 3 | ○ | ○ | ○ | ○ | ○ | 23 | ○ | ○ | ○ | ○ | ○ |
| 4 | ○ | ○ | ○ | ○ | ○ | 24 | ○ | ○ | ○ | ○ | ○ |
| 5 | ○ | ○ | ○ | ○ | ○ | 25 | ○ | ○ | ○ | ○ | ○ |
| 6 | ○ | ○ | ○ | ○ | ○ | 26 | ○ | ○ | ○ | ○ | ○ |
| 7 | ○ | ○ | ○ | ○ | ○ | 27 | ○ | ○ | ○ | ○ | ○ |
| 8 | ○ | ○ | ○ | ○ | ○ | 28 | ○ | ○ | ○ | ○ | ○ |
| 9 | ○ | ○ | ○ | ○ | ○ | 29 | ○ | ○ | ○ | ○ | ○ |
| 10 | ○ | ○ | ○ | ○ | ○ | 30 | ○ | ○ | ○ | ○ | ○ |
| 11 | ○ | ○ | ○ | ○ | ○ | 31 | ○ | ○ | ○ | ○ | ○ |
| 12 | ○ | ○ | ○ | ○ | ○ | 32 | ○ | ○ | ○ | ○ | ○ |
| 13 | ○ | ○ | ○ | ○ | ○ | 33 | ○ | ○ | ○ | ○ | ○ |
| 14 | ○ | ○ | ○ | ○ | ○ | 34 | ○ | ○ | ○ | ○ | ○ |
| 15 | ○ | ○ | ○ | ○ | ○ | 35 | ○ | ○ | ○ | ○ | ○ |
| 16 | ○ | ○ | ○ | ○ | ○ | 36 | ○ | ○ | ○ | ○ | ○ |
| 17 | ○ | ○ | ○ | ○ | ○ | 37 | ○ | ○ | ○ | ○ | ○ |
| 18 | ○ | ○ | ○ | ○ | ○ | 38 | ○ | ○ | ○ | ○ | ○ |
| 19 | ○ | ○ | ○ | ○ | ○ | 39 | ○ | ○ | ○ | ○ | ○ |
| 20 | ○ | ○ | ○ | ○ | ○ | 40 | ○ | ○ | ○ | ○ | ○ |

# WHMIS 2015 & Infection Control

**1. In a BC long-term care facility, a resident is experiencing sudden bouts of vomiting and diarrhea. To break the chain of infection, what is the most effective way to perform hand hygiene after providing care?**

a. Use an Alcohol-Based Hand Rub (ABHR) with at least 70% alcohol
b. Wash hands thoroughly with antimicrobial soap and running water
c. Put on a fresh pair of gloves over the soiled ones before leaving the room
d. Rinse hands with a diluted bleach solution

**2. You find a spray bottle in the utility room containing a blue liquid, but the label has been torn off and is unreadable. What is the correct procedure?**

a. Smell the liquid carefully to identify if it is glass cleaner
b. Use it only on non-porous surfaces like stainless steel
c. Set it aside and notify your supervisor so it can be properly disposed of
d. Create a handwritten label that says “Blue Cleaner” and continue using it

**3. When removing (doffing) PPE after caring for a resident on contact precautions, which item is typically removed first to prevent self-contamination?**

a. Mask or respirator
b. Goggles or face shield
c. Gloves
d. Gown

**4. You are working in a Victoria-based care home during a declared Norovirus outbreak. You observe a coworker using an Alcohol-Based Hand Rub (ABHR) as they exit a resident's room. Why might this action be considered a "Common Trap" in infection control?**

a. ABHR is only effective if used for a minimum of 60 seconds
b. Norovirus is resistant to alcohol; mechanical hand-washing with soap is required
c. ABHR should only be used before care, never after care
d. The coworker must use an N95 mask before using hand sanitizer

**5. A resident with a known history of MRSA (Methicillin-resistant Staphylococcus aureus) in a wound asks to join the others in the common dining area. According to BC "Routine Practices," how should you manage this?**

a. The resident must remain in their room and eat alone until the MRSA is cleared
b. The resident can join the group if the wound is covered by a clean, dry dressing
c. The resident can join the group only if all other residents wear gloves
d. The resident must wear a surgical mask and gown while in the dining area

## The "No-Lift" Policy

**6. When using a sit-to-stand lift, what is a critical safety requirement for the resident?**

a. The resident must be able to follow simple instructions and bear some weight
b. The resident must be completely unconscious to prevent interference
c. The resident must have at least one arm amputated for the sling to fit
d. The resident must be able to walk 10 metres with-

out assistance

**7. You are working with a coworker to move a resident up in bed using a slider sheet. To protect your back and follow safe body mechanics, you should:**

a. Keep your feet together and bend at the waist
b. Twist your torso while pulling the sheet toward the headboard
c. Keep your back straight, knees slightly bent, and shift your weight
d. Hold your breath to create internal pressure and stability

**8. In BC, a "Minimal Assistance" transfer typically means the care provider exerts no more than how much force?**

a. 5 kg (11 lbs)
b. 16 kg (35 lbs)
c. 50 kg (110 lbs)
d. Zero force; the HCA only watches

**9. You are performing a mechanical lift transfer alone. As you begin to raise the resident, the lift makes a loud clicking sound and the motor stops. The resident is suspended 10 cm above the bed. What is your first priority?**

a. Quickly grab the resident and manually pull them onto the bed
b. Leave the room to find a maintenance worker immediately
c. Use the manual emergency lowering release to safely lower the resident
d. Shake the lift to see if the battery connection is just loose

**10. You observe a coworker performing a manual "Axilla Lift" (lifting under the armpits) on a resident who has fallen. Why is this considered a "Common Trap" and a violation of BC safety standards?**

a. It is only allowed if the resident is a family member
b. It can cause serious shoulder or nerve injury to the resident and back injury to the HCA
c. It is the most efficient way to move someone and should be encouraged
d. It is only a violation if the resident complains about pain afterward

## Indigenous Cultural Safety and Humility

**11. In BC healthcare, "Cultural Safety" is best defined as:**

a. A set of facts an HCA memorizes about Indigenous history
b. An outcome where the client feels safe and respected, as defined by the client
c. A policy that requires all staff to speak an Indigenous language
d. The process of treating every client exactly the same regardless of their background

**12. Which BC organization is the primary authority for providing health services and advocacy specifically for First Nations people in the province?**

a. WorkSafeBC
b. First Nations Health Authority (FNHA)
c. BC Care Aide Registry
d. Ministry of Social Development

**13. An Indigenous Elder in a long-term care home keeps a small bundle of dried sage and cedar on their bedside table. While cleaning the room, you should:**

a. Dispose of the dried plants as they are a fire hazard and look like debris
b. Move them to a sealed plastic bag in the closet to keep the room tidy
c. Leave the items in place and treat them with respect as sacred medicines
d. Replace them with a synthetic air freshener to improve the room's scent

**14. During a morning check, a First Nations resident mentions they would like to use a traditional plant-based tea for their cough. As a BC HCA, what is your first responsibility?**

a. Tell the resident that traditional teas are not allowed in the facility
b. Provide the tea immediately because you want to be culturally humble
c. Listen with respect and report the request to the nurse (LPN/RN) to ensure it is safely integrated into the care plan
d. Ignore the request because it is not part of the Western medical doctor's orders

**15. You are helping an Indigenous resident who has many family members visiting at once. The facility has a "two visitors at a time" rule. How should you apply the principle of "Cultural Humility" here?**

a. Strictly enforce the rule and ask the extra family members to leave the building immediately
b. Acknowledge the importance of family (community) in Indigenous wellness and consult your supervisor to find a larger space for the visit
c. Tell the resident they are being disruptive to the other residents
d. Pretend you don't see the visitors so you don't have to deal with the conflict

**16. An Orthodox Jewish resident is served a meal that includes a cheeseburger (meat and dairy together). The resident refuses to eat. Why is this likely a "Common Trap" for a new HCA?**

a. The resident is being difficult and wants a different type of cheese
b. The resident follows Kosher laws which prohibit mixing meat and dairy products in the same meal
c. The resident is likely experiencing a sudden loss of appetite due to illness
d. The resident is waiting for a family member to feed them

**17. While providing care for a resident from a culture that values "high-context" communication, you notice they rarely say "no" directly, even when they seem uncomfortable. To ensure person-centred care, you should:**

a. Assume "yes" always means they are completely satisfied with the care
b. Look for non-verbal cues like body tension or facial expressions and ask clarifying questions gently
c. Speak more loudly to make sure they understand the consequences of their choices
d. Document that the resident is always compliant and has no concerns

**18. A resident's family brings in a traditional herbal remedy from a local community market. They ask you to apply it to the resident's dry skin. What is the safest response?**

a. Apply it immediately as a gesture of cultural safety and respect
b. Read the ingredients and decide yourself if it is safe to use
c. Thank the family for their input and report the request to the nurse to ensure there are no contra indications with the care plan
d. Tell the family that "outside" products are strictly forbidden in BC facilities

**19. You are assisting a resident who practices Buddhism. They have a small altar with a statue of Buddha in their room. You need to clear the bedside table to perform a sterile dressing change. What is the most culturally safe way to handle this?**

a. Move the statue to the floor temporarily to keep the table clear
b. Ask the resident or family for permission and guidance on how to properly move the sacred object
c. Place a towel over the statue so it doesn't get dirty during the procedure
d. Tell the resident that religious items must be kept in the chapel, not the bedroom

**20. During a facility-wide celebration, you notice a resident from a minority culture sitting alone and appearing distressed by the loud music and Western-style food. How should you apply the principle of "The Diverse Mosaic" here?**

a. Encourage them to "join the fun" so they feel more integrated into Canadian culture
b. Acknowledge that the celebration may not reflect their traditions and offer them a quiet space or an alternative activity that feels safe
c. Ignore the resident since they have the right to sit alone if they choose
d. Tell the supervisor that the resident is being "anti-social" during a group activity

## Observation and Reporting

**21. You notice that a resident's urine in their drainage bag is much darker than usual and has a strong, foul odour. How should this be reported?**

a. It doesn't need to be reported unless the resident complains of pain
b. Report the change in colour and odour to the nurse as soon as possible
c. Throw the urine away and wait to see if the next bag looks better
d. Tell the dietary department to increase the resident's juice intake

**22. When documenting an observation in a resident's permanent record, which of the following entries follows BC professional standards?**

a. Resident was a real pain during her bath this morning
b. Resident refused bath; stated "I'm too tired today." LPN notified
c. I think the resident is getting depressed because she cried twice
d. Resident drank a lot of water during the afternoon shift

**23. You are caring for a resident with diabetes. You notice they are sweating profusely, trembling, and appearing unusually irritable. What is the "Common Trap" in this scenario?**

a. Assuming they are just angry because the dining room is late opening
b. Reporting the sweating to the nurse immediately as a sign of hypoglycemia
c. Giving them a sugar-free candy to help them calm down
d. Taking their blood pressure yourself before calling for help

**24. During a transfer, a resident who is usually steady on their feet becomes suddenly weak on one side of their body and their speech becomes slurred. What is your immediate priority?**

a. Finish the transfer to the chair so they are safe and comfortable
b. Call for help immediately and stay with the resident, as these are signs of a stroke
c. Go to the nursing station to find the resident's chart to check for a history of stroke
d. Ask the resident to smile and squeeze your hands to see if they are joking

**25. An HCA is reporting a resident's skin condition to the LPN. Which report provides the most "high-validity" information for the care team?**

a. There is a red spot on his back that looks pretty bad
b. He has a 3 cm non-blanchable reddened area on his coccyx; skin is intact
c. His skin is starting to break down because he won't let me turn him
d. I put some cream on a sore spot I found on his hip earlier this morning

## Documentation "Do's and Don'ts

**26. When you make an error in a paper-based progress note, what is the "BC standard" for correcting it?**

a. Scribble it out until the text is unreadable
b. Use a heavy black marker to cover the mistake
c. Draw a single line through the error, write "void" or "error," and initial it
d. Discard the entire page and start over to keep the chart clean

**27. A resident tells you, "I hate it here and the food**

**is poison." How should you document this subjective statement?**

a. Resident is being paranoid and hates the facility
b. Resident stated, "I hate it here and the food is poison."
c. Resident is refusing to eat because they think the food is bad
d. Resident had a bad attitude during the lunch service

**28. Review this "sloppy" note: "Resident had a large BM. It looked normal. He seems to feel better now." What is the "Common Trap" for a new HCA in this documentation?**

a. Mentioning the size of the BM
b. Using vague, non-descriptive words like "normal" and "seems to feel better"
c. Documenting that the resident had a BM at all
d. Failing to list the exact time the BM occurred

**29. Which of the following notes is the most "high-validity" for a care team monitoring a wound?**

a. The sore on the heel is getting worse and looks gross
b. Applied some lotion to the red spot on the heel as requested by the resident
c. Reddened area on right heel measures 2 cm x 2 cm; no drainage noted. LPN informed
d. The resident's heel is still red; I think they need better shoes

**30. An HCA documents: "Gave the resident her morning meds because the nurse was busy." Why is this a major "Don't" in BC healthcare?**

a. It is too honest about the nurse being busy
b. It documents an action that is outside the HCA's legal scope of practice
c. It doesn't list which specific medications were given
d. It should have been written in the communication book instead of the chart

## Palliative & End-of-Life Care

**31. A Health Care Assistant is asked by a physician to help "set up the room" by bringing in a tray of medical supplies specifically for a MAiD procedure. How should the HCA respond?**

a. Perform the task as it falls under general environmental prep
b. Refuse, as HCAs cannot be involved in any preparation for MAiD
c. Ask a fellow HCA to do it instead to avoid the ethical dilemma
d. Check with the nurse first to ensure the task doesn't cross into "assisting with the procedure"

**32. You are caring for a palliative resident who is becoming increasingly confused. The family asks you to help the resident sign a request for MAiD because "it's what he would have wanted." What is the correct action?**

a. Help steady the resident's hand so they can sign the document clearly
b. Refuse and explain that the resident must have the capacity to provide informed consent
c. Sign as a witness yourself to help the family find peace

d. Immediately notify the nurse of the family's request and the resident's status

**33. Which of the following best describes the "Right of Conscientious Objection" for a health care provider in BC?**

a. You can refuse to provide any care (including feeding or bathing) to a MAiD patient
b. You can refuse to participate in the MAiD process but must continue to provide standard care and respect
c. You must participate if you are the only HCA on shift
d. You can only object if you have a written note from a religious leader

**34. A resident is scheduled for MAiD in two hours. They are experiencing significant breakthrough pain and ask you for their "palliative PRN" (as-needed. medication. What is the most appropriate step?**

a. Withhold the medication so they remain clear-headed for the procedure
b. Tell them they must wait for the MAiD doctor to arrive to get any relief
c. Report the pain to the nurse immediately so comfort medication can be administered
d. Give the medication yourself if it is a simple oral tablet to save time

**35. After a MAiD procedure has been completed, you are assigned to provide post-mortem care. You feel personally conflicted about the procedure. How should you proceed?**

a. Leave the body alone and tell the next shift to handle it
b. Provide the post-mortem care with the same dignity and respect as any other resident
c. Ask the family to perform the post-mortem care

themselves
d. Talk loudly about your objections in the hallway so others know your stance

**36. A resident is "exit-seeking" and follows a staff member toward the keypad-operated door. Which redirection technique is most effective and least restrictive?**

a. Shouting "Stop!" loudly to startle the resident into staying put
b. Walking the resident to a quiet area and offering a favorite snack or activity
c. Grabbing the resident's arm to lead them back to the lounge
d. Turning off the lights in the hallway so the resident can't see the door

**37. You notice a resident who usually wanders calmly is now pacing rapidly, face flushed, and breathing heavily. What should be your first thought?**

a. The resident is just getting their daily exercise
b. The resident may have an unmet physical need, such as pain, hunger, or a need to use the washroom
c. The resident is being intentionally difficult to get attention
d. The resident needs an immediate sedative from the nurse

**38. Which environmental change can help reduce "exit-seeking" behaviour in a dementia care unit without using physical barriers?**

a. Placing a "Stop" sign or a dark mat on the floor in front of the exit
b. Keeping the television on a high volume to drown out outside noises
c. Leaving the exit doors wide open so they don't look like "traps"
d. Using bright, flashing lights near the emergency exits

**39. A resident is highly agitated and insists on leaving to "save my dog." You have tried redirection and validated their feelings, but they are now pushing against you. What is the most appropriate next step?**

a. Use a "team hold" to move the resident to a seclusion room
b. Give the resident a "time out" by locking them in their bedroom
c. Step back to ensure your own safety and immediately notify the nurse of the escalating situation
d. Agree with the resident and tell them you will go get the dog right now if they go to sleep

**40. A family member sees their mother pacing during a sundowning episode and asks, "Why don't you just give her a pill to make her relax or use a bed rail to keep her safe?" How should the HCA explain the BC approach to care?**

a. Tell them that medication and bed rails are too expensive for the facility
b. Explain that we use "least-restraint" policies to maintain dignity and that pacing is a way for her to communicate a need
c. Inform them that law enforcement forbids the use of any medication in care homes
d. Agree with them and say you will ask the doctor for a "chemical restraint" immediately

# The BC Registry Decoder Answers and Analysis

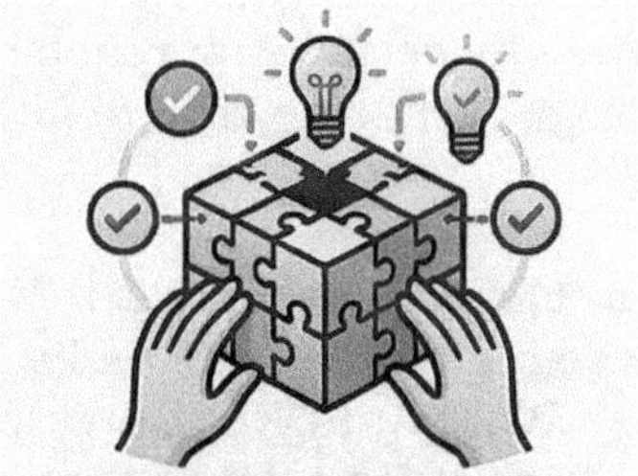

The BC Registry Decoder Answers and Analysis

**Thinking Like a BC Professional**
Welcome to the "Expert" level of your study. If you've just finished these BC-specific questions, you probably noticed that the language shifted. We've moved away from general "good ideas" and into the specific Mandates and Competencies that the BC Ministry of Health and the Care Aide Registry expect from you every single day.

In this section, we aren't just looking at the "right" answer—we're looking at the "Provincially Approved" answer. These rationales are designed to help you "decode" the regulations and see how they apply when you're actually standing at the bedside.

**How to Use the Decoder:**

**The Scope of Practice Filter:** In British Columbia, the line between an HCA and an LPN is very clear. If you got a question wrong about a task (like wound care or medication), read the rationale carefully. It explains exactly where your "Independent" role ends and where "Supervision" or "Delegation" begins.

**The WorkSafeBC Lens:** Many of the "Correct" answers here are dictated by provincial safety laws. If a rationale mentions a Point of Care Risk Assessment (PCRA), pay close attention. That is a term you will use during every single shift once you're on the ward.

**Cultural Safety & Humility:** You likely saw questions regarding Indigenous cultural safety. In BC, this is a core competency, not an "extra." Our rationales explain why certain approaches are required to provide respectful, safe care to all members of our community.

**A Note from the Kitchen Table:**
Some of these regulations can feel a bit like "alphabet soup"—FHA, FOIPPA, PCRA. Don't let the acronyms get to you. These rules exist to protect you just as much as they protect the resident. When you follow the BC Standards, you're covered, you're professional, and you're providing the best care in the country.

## Answers and Analysis

**1. B**
When dealing with C. difficile or Norovirus (indicated by vomiting/diarrhea), alcohol does not kill the spores/virus. Physical friction with soap and water is required.

Option A is the "Common Trap"—ABHR is usually great, but not for these specific "bugs." Option C is a cross-contamination nightmare. Option D is unsafe for skin.

**2. C**
An unlabeled container is a "mystery chemical" and a WHMIS violation. It must be taken out of service immediately.

Option A is dangerous (inhalation risk). Options B and D are major safety violations.

**3. C**
Gloves are considered the most contaminated piece of PPE and are removed first to ensure the hands don't transfer pathogens to the face while removing the mask or goggles.

Options A, B and  are removed after the gloves to protect the mucous membranes.

**4. B**

This is a classic BC exam question. Alcohol sanitizers are the “gold standard” for most things, but they fail against Norovirus and C. diff.

Option A is incorrect (20-30 seconds is standard). Option C is wrong because ABHR is used both before and after.

**5. B**

Routine Practices emphasize that if a “bug” like MRSA is contained (e.g., in a dressed wound. and the resident has good hygiene, they do not need to be isolated from social activities.

Option B is unnecessary isolation and harmful to mental health. Option c and d are “over-precipitating” and not supported by BC health standards.

## The "No-Lift" Policy

**6. A**

A sit-to-stand lift requires the resident to be able to bear weight through their legs and follow the instruction to hold the handles.

Option B is a contraindication (safety risk). Option C is irrelevant. Option D would mean they don’t need a lift.

**7. C**

Good body mechanics in BC training emphasize a wide base of support, using the legs (shifting weight), and keeping the spine neutral (no twisting).

Options A and B describe the exact movements that cause MSIs. Option D (holding breath) can lead to fainting or strain.

**8. B**

Industry standards (Fraser Health, Interior Health) often

cite a 15.9 kg or roughly 16 kg (35 lbs) limit for "minimal assistance" under ideal conditions.

Option A is too low for most tasks. Option C is far too high (manual lifting). Option D is "independent," not "minimal assistance."

**9. C**

All mechanical lifts in BC must have an emergency manual release. This is the safest way to return a resident to a surface if the power fails.

Option A risks a fall/injury. Option B leaves the resident in a dangerous position. Option D is unsafe while the resident is suspended.

**10. B**

Manual lifts using the axilla (armpit) are strictly prohibited in BC as they are high-risk for both the HCA and the resident.

This is the "Common Trap." It feels like a natural way to help, but it is one of the most common causes of worker injury and resident skin tears/dislocations.

## Indigenous Cultural Safety and Humility

**11. B**

Cultural Safety is an outcome. It is not about the HCA's intent; it is about whether the person receiving care feels safe. This is defined by the client.

Option A is "Cultural Awareness." Option C is a misconception. Option D ("treating everyone the same") is actually "Cultural Blindness," which can be harmful.

**12. B**

The First Nations Health Authority (FNHA. is unique to BC and is the first province-wide health authority of its kind in Canada.

WorkSafeBC (Choice A. is for workplace safety. The Registry (Choice C. is for staff regulation.

**13. C**

Sage, cedar, sweetgrass, and tobacco are the four sacred medicines for many Indigenous peoples. They are often used for protection and wellness.

Tossing them (Choice A. or hiding them (Choice b. is a violation of the resident's spiritual rights and a sign of cultural disrespect.

**14. C**

Respecting traditional medicine means recognizing its value while ensuring safety. HCAs must work within the care team (reporting to the LPN/RN) to check for drug-plant interactions.

Option A is culturally unsafe. Option B is out of scope (HCA cannot authorize new treatments).

**15. B**

In many Indigenous cultures, wellness is communal, not just individual. Humility involves being flexible with "Western" rules to support a resident's spirit.

Strictly enforcing rules (Choice A. without looking for a solution can create a "racist or discriminatory" experience for the family.

**16. B**

This is the "Common Trap." A student might think the resident is picky, but under Kosher laws, mixing meat and milk in the same meal (or even on the same plate) is forbidden.

Options A, C and D are medical or behavioural assumptions that ignore the cultural context of the food itself.

**17. B**

In high-context cultures, direct confrontation is often avoided to maintain "harmony." The HCA must use active observation to ensure the resident's needs are truly being met.

Option A is a dangerous assumption. Option C is aggressive. Option D ignores the HCA's duty to provide accurate observations.

**18. C**

Even "natural" or "traditional" products can have active ingredients that interfere with medications or cause skin reactions. Everything must be vetted by the nurse/care plan.

Option A is a safety risk. Option B is out of the HCA's scope of practice.

**19. B**

In many cultures, placing a sacred object on the floor is a major sign of disrespect. Asking for guidance shows "Cultural Humility."

Option A is a cultural insult. Option C is well-meaning but doesn't address the placement. Option D is a violation of the right to express spirituality in one's own living space.

**20. B**

Inclusion isn't about forcing everyone to do the same thing; it's about making sure everyone has a way to feel comfortable and respected.

Option A is "Cultural Assimilation." Option D uses negative labeling for a valid cultural or personal response to an environment.

## Observation and Reporting

**21. B**

Changes in urine characteristics are significant observations that can indicate dehydration or infection.

Ignoring it (Choice A. or discarding evidence (Choice C. prevents diagnosis. Giving juice (Choice D. is a dietary intervention outside the HCA's scope.

**22. B**

Documentation must be objective, use quotes for subjective statements, and indicate what action was taken (notifying the nurse).

Option A is judgmental. Option C is an interpretation. Option D is too vague ("a lot" is not a measurement).

**23. B**

Sweating, trembling, and irritability are signs of low blood sugar (hypoglycemia). This is a medical emergency that requires immediate reporting.
The "Common Trap" (Choice A. is dismissing physical symptoms as "behavioural" or mood-related. Option C is dangerous (sugar-free won't help). Option D is often outside the entry-level scope during an emergency.

**24. D**

Sudden one-sided weakness and slurred speech are hallmarks of a stroke. The HCA must stay with the resident to prevent falls and call for immediate help.

Completing the transfer (Choice A. could be dangerous if the resident collapses. Leaving the room (Choice C. is unsafe. Joking (Choice D. wastes critical "Time is Brain" minutes.

**25. B**

This report uses specific measurements, anatomical locations, and clinical terms (non-blanchable) that help the nurse assess the stage of a pressure injury.

Option A is too vague. Option C is blaming and non-descriptive. Option D describes an unauthorized intervention (applying cream to a new wound without a plan).

💡 **Test Tip:** When a question asks for a "Priority Action" regarding a change of status, look for the answer that involves reporting to the nurse immediately.

## Documentation "Do's and Don'ts

**26. C**
This is the legal standard for medical charting in Canada. It ensures the original text is still visible, maintaining the integrity of the record.

Scribbling (Choice A. or blacking out (Choice b. looks like you are trying to hide something. Tearing out pages (d. is illegal in many jurisdictions.

**27. B**
When documenting subjective statements, use the resident's exact words in quotation marks.

Options A, C and D all add the HCA's interpretation to the resident's words.

**28. B**
Explanation: The "Common Trap" is using "filler" words. "Normal" means different things to different people. A better note would describe colour and consistency.

Why Distractors are Wrong: Documenting BMs (c. is a standard HCA task. While time (d. is important, the lack of description is the primary error here.

**29. C**
This note provides objective measurements and indicates that the proper authority (LPN) was told.

"Gross" (Choice A. is unprofessional. Applying lotion (Choice b. without a nurse's order for a wound is unsafe. "Better shoes" (Choice D. is an HCA's guess, not a clinical observation.

**30. B**
In BC, HCAs do not "give" (administer) medications. This is a regulated task for nurses. Documenting that you performed a task outside your scope is a massive legal risk.

The main issue isn't the "busyness" or the lack of detail; it's the violation of the scope of practice.

## Palliative & End-of-Life Care

**31. D**

This is a grey area. Setting up a room is generally fine, but the HCA should ensure they aren't inadvertently assisting in the medical preparation of the drugs or specialized equipment.

Choice B is incorrect; it is too extreme. HCAs still maintain the resident's environment.

**32. D**

MAiD requires "Informed Consent" at the time of the request and immediately before the procedure. An HCA cannot facilitate a signature, especially if capacity is in question.

Choice A is incorrect; this is a major legal and ethical violation.

Choice B is incorrect; while true, the HCA should report to the nurse rather than just giving a lecture to the family.

**33. B**

Providers have the right to not participate in the MAiD procedure itself, but they cannot abandon the resident's basic care needs.

Choice A is incorrect; refusing basic care is considered abandonment/neglect.

**34. C**

Comfort care does not stop because MAiD is scheduled. Pain management remains a priority until the very end.

Choice A is incorrect; withholding pain relief is unethical.

Common Trap: Option A. Students often think "clear-headedness" for the final consent means the resident must suffer in pain.

**35. B**
Professionalism requires that we treat every resident with dignity after death, regardless of the circumstances of that death.

Choices A and C are incorrect as they constitute a failure to perform job duties.

**Test Tip:** On the BC HCA exam, whenever a resident asks for something "medical" or "legal," the correct answer almost always involves reporting to the regulated nurse or providing comfort while staying within your scope. If an answer choice has you giving "advice" or "opinions," it's usually the wrong path.

## Mental Health & Cognitive Impairment

**36. B**
This is the least restrictive and most person-centred approach.

Choice D is a Common Trap. While "hiding" a door with shadows is a trick sometimes used, turning off lights can increase the risk of falls and heighten fear/confusion.

**37. B**
In BC HCA training, "Behaviour is Communication." If a resident's baseline changes, look for a physical cause first.

Choice D is incorrect; medication should be a last resort after searching for the root cause.

**38. A**
A dark mat often looks like a "hole" or a "gap" to someone with altered depth perception from dementia, discouraging them from stepping on it.

Choice B is incorrect; loud noise (over-stimulation) usually increases agitation.

**39. C**

Safety first. If redirection fails and the resident becomes physically aggressive, you must create space and get clinical support.

Choice D is incorrect; "therapeutic lying" should be used carefully, but promising to do something impossible (getting a dog) can lead to a loss of trust when the promise isn't kept.

**40. B**

This reflects the BC Ministry of Health's "Least Restraint" guidelines.

Choice D is a Common Trap. "Chemical restraint" is a real term, but it is a negative one that facilities work hard to avoid.

**Test Tip:** On the HCA exam, if you see an answer that involves "Reminding the resident they are in a care home" or "Correcting their memory," it is usually the wrong answer. Look for options that involve "Validation," "Redirection," and "Safety."

# BC Care Aide Career Roadmap

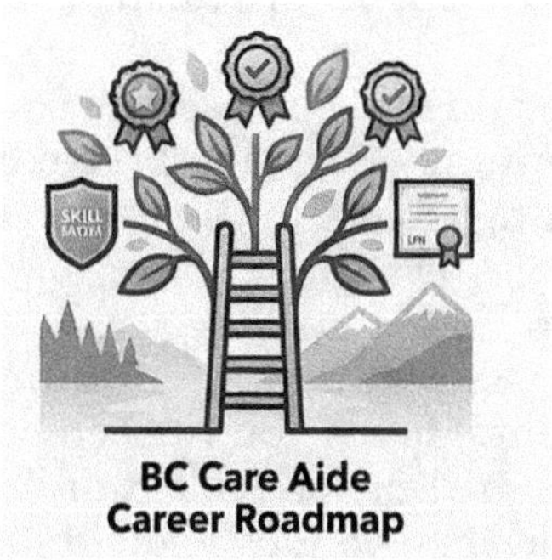


**Welcome to the Front Lines: Your BC Care Aide Career Roadmap!**

If you're holding this workbook, it means you've decided to step up for your community. Whether you're at a kitchen table in Saanich, a coffee shop in Prince George, or a library in Vancouver, I want to start by saying: Thank you. In the big world of healthcare, the "Big Prep" companies tend to focus on the doctors and the high-level administrators. But here at our small office in Victoria, we know the truth—the Care Aide is the heart of the system. You are the one who knows the residents best. You see the small changes in their health, you provide the comfort, and you uphold the dignity of our seniors every single day.

But passing the BC HCA exam is just the first door. This roadmap is here to help you see what lies beyond that door.

**Beyond the Exam**

In British Columbia, we have a unique and rewarding healthcare landscape. Once you've secured your spot on the BC Care Aide & Community Health Worker Registry, you aren't just a "worker"—you are a professional with a path.

**This roadmap is designed to show you:**

**The Environments:** The difference between working in a bustling Health Authority hospital versus a quiet, private assisted-living home.

**The Specializations:** How to move into specialized areas like Mental Health support or Palliative care.

**The Ladder:** How this role can serve as a rock-solid foundation if you eventually decide to bridge into Nursing (LPN or RN) programs right here in the Pacific Northwest.

**Why We Do This**

At Complete Test Preparation, we've always been for the "forgotten" student. Maybe you've been out of school for twenty years. Maybe English isn't your first language. Maybe you're working two jobs while trying to study.

We don't just want you to pass a test; we want you to have a career that pays the bills, offers a pension, and gives you a sense of pride when you head home at the end of a shift.

You've got the heart for this job. We're just here to give you the tools and the map.

**Let's get to work.**

# The BC Care Aide Regulatory Cheat Sheet

**Your Map to the BC Registry & Core Competencies**
Welcome to the profession. In British Columbia, being a Care Aide isn't just a job; it's a regulated role overseen by the BC Care Aide & Community Health Worker Registry. To get your CA number and stay in good standing, you need to master the Core Competencies set by the Ministry of Health.

**The "Big Three" BC Pillars**
In BC, every question on your exam and every task at the bedside is filtered through these three lenses. If you're stuck on a practice question, ask yourself: "Which answer best supports these three things?"

**1. Person-Centred Care**

**The BC Standard:** You aren't just "treating a patient"; you are supporting a person.

**The "Cheat":** Always look for the answer that respects the resident's choice, history, and dignity. If the resident wants to wear the blue shirt instead of the red one, the "BC way" is to let them choose.

**2. Safety & Assisted Living Standards**

**The BC Standard:** We have strict provincial guidelines on falls prevention, infection control (especially post-pandemic), and safe body mechanics.

**The "Cheat":** If a question involves a lift or a transfer, the answer is always "Safety First." No shortcuts, no "doing it alone" if the care plan says two people.

**3. Collaborative Practice**

**The BC Standard:** You are the "eyes and ears" for the LPNs and RNs.

**The "Cheat":** Questions about "what to do next" often lead to Reporting and Recording. In BC, if you didn't document it, it didn't happen.

## Mapping the BC HCA Landscape: Where Will You Work?

Passing your exam is the "ticket" to the show, but you still have to decide which stage you want to stand on. In British Columbia, the employer you choose—and the union that backs them—dictates your lifestyle.

| Feature | Health Authorities (e.g., Island Health, VCH) | Private Assisted Living | Home Support (Public& Private) |
|---|---|---|---|
| Typical Setting | Hospitals & Public Long-Term Care | Private Seniors' Residences | Client's Private Homes |
| Primary Union | HEU (Facilities Agreement) | Various (or Non-Union) | BCGEU or HEU |
| Starting Pay (2026) | Approx. \$28.50 - \$30.00/hr | Can vary widely (\$23 - \$29/hr) | \$27.00 - \$29.00/hr |
| Pension | Municipal Pension Plan (The Gold Standard) | Rare (usually RRSP matching) | Depends on the agency |

| | | | |
|---|---|---|---|
| Sick Days | Up to 18 days/year (fully vested) | Often the BC minimum (5 days) | Varies by collective agreement |

**1. The "Roadmap" Insider:** Unions and Agreements
In BC, most Care Aides in the public sector are covered by the Facilities Bargaining Association (FBA), led by the HEU.

**The Big Win:** As of late 2025/2026, the BC government has been moving thousands of private care-home workers back into the "public" agreement. This is great news for you—it means more sites now offer the same high wages and "portable" benefits.

**The "Brian" Tip:** If you move from a job at Victoria General (Island Health) to a public care home in Nanaimo, your seniority and pension usually follow you. That's the power of the provincial agreement.

**2. Decoding the Job Postings:** Casual vs. Permanent
When you look at the Island Health or Fraser Health job boards, you'll see these terms. Here's what they actually mean for your kitchen-table budget:

**Casual (The "Foot in the Door"):** Most new grads start here. You don't have a set schedule; you "pick up" shifts.

**The Upside:** You get an extra 12-13% "pay in lieu" of benefits. Your hourly rate looks huge, but you don't get paid vacation or dental.

**Permanent Part-Time/Full-Time (The "Line"):** This is a "line" on the schedule. You know exactly when you work.

**The Upside:** Stability. You get the full benefits package (medical, dental, and pension). For most people, this is the goal for long-term career health.

**3. The "Roadmap" Strategy**
If you're just starting out, don't be afraid of Casual roles. In BC, "Casual" Care Aides often work 40 hours a week because the demand is so high. It's a great way to "test drive" different wards—try Dementia care for a week, then try Acute care—before you commit to a permanent line.

**A Note from the Kitchen Table:**
When you're looking at a job offer, don't just look at the hourly wage. A private facility might offer you $31/hr but no pension. A Health Authority job might offer $29.50/hr but with a pension that pays you for the rest of your life. In the long run, the "public" route usually wins.

## Navigating the Registry: Your First 90 Days

You've studied hard and you're ready for the floor. But before you can put on those scrubs for a BC Health Authority, you need to navigate the "Registry Maze." Think of this as your professional licensing board.

Here is your step-by-step checklist to get from "Student" to "Registered HCA."

**Step 1: The "Paperwork" Push (Days 1–10)**

As soon as you finish your program, don't wait for your graduation ceremony.

- **The Task:** Apply online at cachwr.bc.ca.
- **What you need:** An official transcript or a "Letter of Completion" from your school.
- **The "Brian" Tip:** Use a desktop computer for this, not your phone. The Registry website is notoriously picky about file attachments, and a laptop makes it much easier to upload your transcripts without the system crashing.

**Step 2: The ID & Criminal Record Check (Days 10–30)**

This is where most students get stuck. You have to undergo a **Criminal Record Review Program (CRRP)** check specifically for "Vulnerable Adults."

- **The Task:** You'll receive an "Access Code" from the Registry once your initial application is reviewed. Use this code on the BC Government's Justice website.

- **The Identity Secret:** The fastest way to do this is using your **BC Services Card app**. If you don't have the app set up on your phone yet, do it now. It turns a 3-week waiting period into a 5-minute online verification.

**Step 3: The Competency Confirmation (Days 30–60)**

The Registry needs to know you didn't just "pass"—they need to know you are safe.

- **The Task:** If you are a new grad from a BC program, your school usually sends a "Graduate Verification List" directly to the Registry.
- **The Follow-up:** Don't assume they sent it. Check in with your program coordinator two weeks after your last clinical shift to ensure your name was on that list.

**Step 4: The HCA Number (Days 60–90)**

Once the Registry has your transcripts, your cleared criminal record check, and your school's verification, they will move your status to **"ACTIVE."**

- **The Prize:** You will be issued a **Registration Number (HCA Number)**.
- **The Roadmap Link:** This number is exactly what HR at Island Health or Vancouver Coastal will ask for. Write it down, memorize it, and put it at the very top of your resume.

**Registry "Red Flags" to Avoid**

- **The Name Gap:** If your ID says "Robert" but your school transcript says "Bob," the Registry will pause your application for weeks. Make sure your name is identical on every single document.
- **The $28 Fee:** The Criminal Record Check usually costs about $28. It's the only fee you'll likely pay (registration itself is currently free!), so have a credit card ready so you don't delay the process.
- **The Lapse:** You have to "renew" your status every year. It's free, but if you forget, you disappear from the employer's database. Mark your calendar for your registration anniversary!

## The BC "Gold Standard": Dementia & Cognitive Care

The reality of healthcare in the Pacific Northwest is that our population is aging. Whether you're in a hospital or home support, a huge percentage of your residents will be living with some form of dementia.

**The Skill:** Look for GPA (Gentle Persuasive Approaches) or P.I.E.C.E.S. training.

**Why it makes you valuable:** It's about more than just patience. These certifications teach you the "why" behind challenging behaviors. When you can de-escalate a situation with a calm word and a specific technique, the whole floor runs smoother. You become the person everyone looks to when things get tough.

**2. Palliative and End-of-Life Care**
Providing comfort to someone—and their family—during their final days is perhaps the most sacred part of our job.

**The Skill:** The BC Hospice Palliative Care Association (BCHPCA. offers workshops specifically for Health Care Assistants.

**Why it makes you valuable:** It's a specialized kind of "soft skill." Knowing how to provide physical comfort (mouth care, positioning) and emotional support during the active dying phase makes you an indispensable part of a palliative team.

**3. Advanced Skin Care & Pressure Ulcer Prevention**
In long-term care, skin is everything.

**The Skill: Take a weekend workshop on Wound Care Prevention.**

**Why it makes you valuable:** While the Nurse handles

the dressings, you are the one doing the bathing and the dressing. If you are the person who notices a tiny "stage one" redness on a resident's heel before it be**comes a ma**jor problem, you've just saved that resident months of pain. That kind of sharp eye is worth its weight in gold to a Charge Nurse.

**4. Leadership & Mentoring**
Once you have a year or two under your belt, you'll see new students coming onto the floor looking just as nervous as you feel today.

**The Skill:** Ask about Preceptor Training through your Health Authority (like Island Health's internal programs).

**Why it makes you valuable:** It puts you on the path to becoming a Lead Care Aide. It shows management that you aren't just there to do your tasks—you're there to build the team.

**The "Brian" Pro-Tip: Let the Employer Pay**
Before you reach into your own pocket for a workshop, check your HEU or BCGEU collective agreement. Many of these contracts have "Professional Development" funds.

**Tell your manager:** "I'm really interested in improving my skills in Dementia care. Is there a way the facility can support me in taking a GPA course?" More often than not, they'll jump at the chance to have a more skilled person on the floor.

# The BC Healthcare Staircase: Where Can This Take You?

In the Pacific Northwest, we don't believe in dead-end jobs. Being a Care Aide is a fantastic career in its own right, but for many, it's also the first step on a ladder that leads to nursing, specialized therapy, or healthcare management.

Here is how the "Staircase" usually looks in our province:

**Level 1: Community Health Worker (Home Support)**

- **The Setting:** Visiting clients in their own homes or assisted living suites.
- **The Vibe:** You are independent. You're out in the community, often driving between appointments. You get to see people in their natural environment.
- **Why start here?** It builds incredible communication skills and "street smarts." You learn to be resourceful because you don't have a supply room down the hall.

**Level 2: Facility-Based Care Aide (Long-Term or Acute Care)**

- **The Setting:** Nursing homes (Long-Term Care) or hospitals (Acute Care).
- **The Vibe:** You are part of a fast-paced team. You're working alongside LPNs, RNs, and Doctors.
- **Why move here?** This is where you master the "technical" side of care—complex lifts, monitoring vitals, and working with specialized equipment. In BC, Acute Care (hospital) roles often come with a slight pay premium.

**Level 3: The Specialist (Mental Health, Pediatrics, or Hospice)**

- **The Setting:** Specialized wards, group homes, or the BC Children's Hospital.
- **The Vibe:** You aren't just a "generalist" anymore. You have extra training in areas like Mental Health support or pediatric care.

- **Why aim for this?** It's deeply rewarding work. You become the "go-to" person for specific, sensitive needs. It often leads to more stable, permanent "lines" (schedules) because your skills are harder to replace.

**Level 4: The Bridge (LPN or RN Programs)**

- **The Setting:** Back to school (Camosun, BCIT, UVic, etc.).
- **The Vibe:** You're using your years of bedside experience to become a Licensed Practical Nurse or Registered Nurse.
- **The "BC Advantage":** Most BC colleges offer "Access" or "Bridge" programs. They recognize your HCA certificate and your work hours, allowing you to skip the basics and finish your nursing degree faster.

**The "Brian" Pro-Tip: The "Earn While You Learn" Secret**

The best part about the BC staircase? You don't have to quit your job to climb it. Because of our strong unions (like the HEU), many Care Aides work "casual" shifts on weekends while they go to nursing school during the week. You keep your seniority, you keep your pension growing, and you have a guaranteed job waiting for you the second you graduate.

**A Note from the Kitchen Table:** Don't feel like you have to rush to Level 4. Some Care Aides in Victoria who have stayed at Level 2 for thirty years because they love the residents and the "hands-on" nature of the work. The beauty of this staircase is that **you** decide when to stop climbing. Every step is a respectable, well-paying career.

## The BC Health Care Career Staircase

| Career Level | Job Title | Required Training for an HCA | Est. Salary (BC 2026) |
|---|---|---|---|
| Level 1 | Community Health Worker | BC HCA Certificate + Registry | $27.00 - $29.00/ hr |
| Level 2 | Acute Care Aide (Hospital) | BC HCA Certificate + Hospital Experience | $29.50 - $31.00/ hr |
| Level 3 | Activity Assistant | HCA Cert + ~4-month Post-Sec Certificate | $30.00 - $31.50/ hr |
| Level 3 | Mental Health Worker | HCA Cert + 15-week Specialist Cert | $31.00 - $33.50/ hr |
| Level 3 | Renal / Dialysis Tech | Employer-paid training (post-hiring) | $31.00 - $32.00/ hr |
| Level 3 | MDRT (Sterilization Tech) | ~4-8 month College Certificate | $29.00 - $31.00/ hr |
| Level 4 | Licensed Practical Nurse | Access to PN Program (approx. 12-14 months) | $32.00 - $38.00/ hr |

www.ingramcontent.com/pod-product-compliance
Lightning Source LLC
LaVergne TN
LVHW022056200926
848481LV00003B/938